VIAGRA

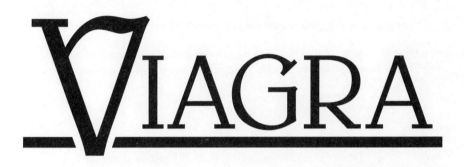

VIAGRA

How the Miracle Drug Happened
& What It Can Do for You!

JONATHAN P. JAROW, M.D.
ROBERT A. KLONER, M.D., PH.D.
ANN M. HOLMES

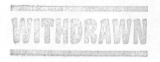

M. EVANS AND COMPANY, INC.
New York

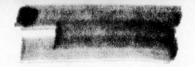

M. Evans and Company, Inc.
216 East 49th Street
New York, New York 10017

Library of Congress Cataloging-in-Publication Data

Jarow, Jonathan.
    Viagra : how the miracle drug happened & what it can do for you! /
Jonathan Jarow, Robert A. Kloner, and Ann M. Holmes.
      p. cm.
    Includes biographical references and index.
    ISBN 0-87131-877-6 (cloth)
    1. Sildenafil—Popular works. 2. Impotence—Chemotherapy.
I. Kloner, Robert A., Anthony. II. Holmes, Ann A. II. Title.
RC889.J36 1998
616.6'92061—dc21   98–39151

Viagra® is a registered trademark of Pfizer Inc.

Design and composition by John Reinhardt Book Design

Manufactured in the United States of America

9 8 7 6 5 4 3 2 1

Contents

Acknowledgments

The authors wish to express their sincere gratitude to Karen Asouty, Emily Donovan, Cathie Eagle, and Ian Hemenway for their editorial support, and most of all to Mrs. Patricia F. Wasserman, without whose consistent encouragement and support this book would not be possible.

Disclaimer

The statements contained in this work are the opinions of the authors. They are not to be deemed expert medical opinions or qualified medical advice. As with any pharmaceutical product or medical procedure, readers are cautioned to consult with their own physician or medical expert before using any drugs or proceeding with any treatment. Use of Viagra may present medical and other risks to some people.(Please see Chapter 7 for "Contraindications and Potential Side Effects of Viagra.") Neither the authors nor the publisher of this work shall be liable for damages (whether actual, incidental, or consequential) arising from the use of Viagra or of any other product or procedure discussed in this work.

All of the names of patients in this book have been changed to protect their anonymity. In addition, to ensure patient privacy, in some instances the authors have combined reports from one or more patients to create a case; however, the details provided in each case are based on actual patient experiences.

1

You Are *Not* Alone!

Yes, Viagra* is new—and news—but impotence isn't. In a society that places a high value on well-toned bodies, virility, robust health, and youth, the inability to perform sexually is a disorder to which very few American men will admit. In fact, in the Catholic church an annulment—the dissolution of a marriage—is granted only in the rarest of circumstances; impotence is one. Across the country, in some states impotence is viewed with such disdain that it is considered grounds for divorce. Still, despite the havoc it wreaks, for centuries major medical research centers around the world have ignored impotence. Incredibly, in fact, impotence—more properly known as erectile dysfunction, or E.D.—is probably the last stigmatized condition to receive recognition and study, decades after menopause, alcoholism, depression, and obsessive-compulsive disorder saw the light of day. Why? Some say the belief that impotence is "all in your head" was enough to keep any serious medical investigation at bay; others believed it was the excruciatingly personal dimension of the disorder that discouraged investigation; still others felt it wasn't a significant problem. Not significant, you say? Well, try this on for size: Worldwide, it is estimated that approximately 100,000,000 men suffer from E.D.—and that's just an estimate! But, unfortunately, even today, less than 10 percent of these men seek treatment.

Specific information about impotence varies from country to country. In China, for example, there were no outpatient clinics for sexual disorders in the mid-1980s but, by 1994, there were thirty-four! In the United

---

*Viagra® is a registered trademark of Pfizer Inc.

1

Figure 1. <u>Prevalence of minimal, moderate, and complete impotence
(The Massachusetts Male Aging Study, 1994)</u>

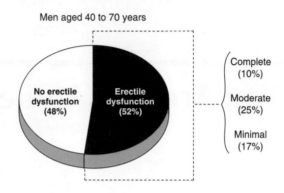

Men aged 40 to 70 years

No erectile dysfunction (48%)

Erectile dysfunction (52%)

Complete (10%)

Moderate (25%)

Minimal (17%)

Adapted with permission from Feldman, H.A., Goldstein, I., Hatzchristou, D.G., Krane, R.J., and McKinlay, J.B. "Impotence and its medical and psychological correlates: results of the Massachusetts Male Aging Study. *J Urol.* 151 (1994) 54–61.

States, a 1985 report from the National Center for Health Statistics revealed that there were approximately 400,000 outpatient visits to physicians, related to impotence, as well as 30,000 hospital admissions. The
total direct cost of the hospital admissions was a whopping $140 mil-
lion! Later, from 1987 to 1989, a large random sample survey of 1,290
noninstitutionalized men, ranging in age from forty to seventy years,
was carried out in eleven cities and towns near Boston, Massachusetts.
Overall, the combined prevalence of minimal, moderate, and complete
impotence was 52 percent (Figure 1). Referred to as the Massachusetts
Male Aging Study (MMAS), the physicians who organized the study concluded that impotence is a "major health concern" that has a substantial
impact on the quality of life in men, especially as they age (Figure 2).
Today, we recognize that erectile dysfunction is, indeed, a common medical problem, but with effective therapy such as Viagra, this disorder can
be treated successfully, and men and their partners can continue to enjoy a fulfilling sexual life.

So, are we the first generation to step up to the plate and try to manage E.D.? Hardly. As far as we know, man's attempts to stave off the scourge

Figure 2. Prevalence of erectile dysfunction increased with age in the Massachusetts Male Aging Study

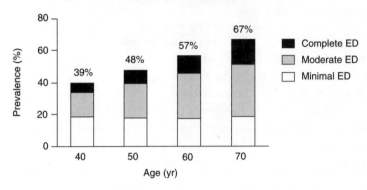

Adapted with permission from Feldman, H.A., Goldstein, I., Hatzchristou, D.G., Krane, R.J., and McKinlay, J.B. "Impotence and its medical and psychological correlates: results of the Massachusetts Male Aging Study. *J Urol.* 151 (1994) 54–61.

of E.D. stretches back thousands of years. Some of the earliest therapeutic approaches ranged from eating a dried centipede to remedy an excessively limp penis to a more palatable approach selected by the early Hindus in India: just drink a cup of fresh grape juice. Ancient Romans also tried to cope with the malady that had diminished men through the ages, resorting to everything from onions to rotting fish. Ovid turned to goose tongue for a remedy, while ancient Egyptians chose the radish. In medieval Italy, the common therapy was rubbing crocodile semen on the genitalia. But in Renaissance France, delicacies were considered the key to unlocking potency. Some men, for example, consumed far more than their fair share of artichokes, while others relied on asparagus to "stir up bodily lust in a man." Caviar and oysters were thought to enhance a man's potency, too. The Aztecs believed in simple, true-blue chocolate—just eat as much as you can per day—while Africans ate the bark of the yohimbine tree, a remedy that is still in use today.

Literature, too, is sprinkled with references to that demonic curse, impotency. In the sixteenth century, for example, Montaigne wrote: "I shall never give impotence thanks for anything it does for me." Well-known

Table 1.

THE AILMENT: IMPOTENCE AND ITS CURES
THROUGH THE AGES

Ancient China	eat dried centipedes
Ancient Rome	eat onions, rotting fish
Ancient Greece	eat goose tongue
India	drink fresh grape juice
Ancient Egypt	eat radishes
Medieval Italy	rub crocodile semen on genitalia
Renaissance France	eat artichokes, asparagus, caviar, and oysters
Aztec Indians	eat lots of chocolate
Africans	eat bark of the yohimbine tree

writers from the sixteenth through the twentiest century addressed it, too. Why such recognition through the ages? Because even the sound of the condition conjures up an image of weakness: impotency. What else does it mean but loss of power? It's no wonder, then that men from the ancient Greeks and Romans on—warriors, soldiers, statesmen, too—searched for a libido "magic bullet" to conquer the ill of ills! Yet, for centuries there was so little progress in both diagnosis and treatment. In fact, up until the 1960s, 95 percent of men who suffered from E.D. (or impotency, as it was called then) were thought to have severe psychopathology. Even the Merck Manual, a desktop "bible" of diseases and treatments for physicians, listed impotency as a psychological disorder as late as 1990! Finally, in the mid-1990s, medical researchers developed compounds for treatment, and, working with different pharmaceutical companies, these treatments became available (see Chapter 7 for more information). For the first time, men with E.D. could get professional medical help and treatment for their condition.

Yet, where are they? In light of what we now know about the prevalence of E.D., it is clear to us that there are still a vast number of men with E.D. who remain reluctant to seek treatment. Still, with the introduction of Viagra and the candor with which everyone from news journalists to television and radio talk show hosts are now discussing Viagra, we hope that more men who need treatment will seek it. To learn more about male erectile dysfunction—its causes and treatment options, simply read on! In addition to this text, which we hope you will consider a valuable resource, you can also consult one of the following organizations for more information:

- Impotence Centers of America (ICA), based in Westfield, New Jersey: 800 515-0005
- Men's Health Centers (Florida only): 800 982-1471

WHAT THE MASSACHUSETTS MALE AGING STUDY TAUGHT US ABOUT IMPOTENCE

The results of an important study were published in the *Journal of Urology* in 1994 in a paper entitled, "Impotence and its Medical and Psychosocial Correlates: Results of the Massachusetts Male Aging Study." The investigators questioned men forty to seventy years old in eleven randomly selected cities and towns in the Boston area. Sexual questionnaires were filled out by 1,290 men who answered questions related to erection and their ability to have an erection. Unlike some previous studies, this one established grades of E.D. by asking men to characterize themselves as "not impotent, minimally impotent, moderately impotent, or completely impotent." This approach was important because the study looked at *grades* of impotence.

An incredible 52 percent of the forty- to seventy-year-old men in the sample claimed some degree of impotence, ranging from complete impotence in only 9.6 percent of the men, to moderate impotence in 25.2 percent, and minimal impotence in 17.2 percent of the men.

In this survey, age was a risk factor for E.D. Whereas complete E.D. was reported in 5.1 percent of forty-year-old men, it increased to 15 percent in seventy-year-old men. Moderate ED, on the other hand, increased from 17% in forty-year-old men to 34% in seventy-year-old men.

Also, after adjusting for age, certain common diseases were significantly associated with E.D.; for example, diabetes, heart disease, and hypertension (high blood pressure). You'll read more about the role these diseases play in E.D. in Chapter 2.

What did the Massachusetts Male Aging Study teach us? To begin with, researchers and practicing physicians alike now realize that the prevalence of impotence, including degrees of impotence, is more common than many of us had thought. Second, we discovered that E.D. correlates with certain risk factors—some we may be able to modify, such as smoking, hypertension, and diabetes, while others we can't change, such as age. Interestingly, this study was also the first to identify a low HDL (high-density lipoprotein) cholesterol as significantly correlated with impotence (see Chapter 2). Lastly, we realized that in order to treat men effectively and appropriately for E.D., we—medical health care professionals—would have to try to help our patients by talking with them about E.D.

2

Male Erectile Dysfunction
What Is It?

By 1993, a National Institutes of Health (NIH) panel comprised of lead-ing urologists, psychiatrists, psychologists, gerontologists (physicians who specialize in aging), and surgeons posed the question: What is male erectile dysfunction? The term "impotence," they found, was sometimes confusing, and they readily acknowledged that labeling a man "impo-tent" often left male patients with a "gloom-and-doom" outlook. Over the course of the meeting, the experts decided to create a more appropri-ate medical term to describe a man's inability to achieve and sustain an erection. They created a more accurate definition of erectile dysfunc-tion: "An inability of the male to achieve an erect penis as part of the overall multifaceted process of male sexual function." This includes not only achieving an erection, but also maintaining an erection for satisfac-tory sexual intercourse. Their report, entitled the NIH Consensus Con-ference Development Panel on Impotence, was published in July 1993, in the highly regarded peer-review medical journal, The *Journal of the American Medical Association*. Prior to this, the term impotence had been used to describe male erectile dysfunction.

And what did the term impotence mean to most of us—men and women—up until very recently?

Even the NIH consensus panel recognized that the term impotence had pejorative implications. It is no wonder, then, that for so long so many men with E.D. chose to hide their problem. Impotence, they felt, was associated with weakness, and/or failure, and feelings of shame. Of

7

course, many just simply felt too embarrassed to seek medical treatment. Instead, for many of these men, their self-esteem was left to erode, feelings of inadequacy prevailed, and, ultimately, the intimate relationship they shared with their partners faltered. Feelings of anxiety, anger, and/or depression were common in these men, too. One of the objectives of the NIH panel, then, was to recognize the significance of this condition, E.D., and call appropriate attention to it as a medical problem. Thus, the panel recommended replacing the term impotence with male erectile dysfunction, or E.D.

Despite the NIH recommendation, however, the term impotence still appears frequently—in medical journal articles, health care magazines, and the consumer press. We believe it is important to foster use of the proper medical description of this disorder, so we will use the term E.D. throughout this book.

When the NIH issued its consensus statement in 1993 on E.D., they noted, among other things, that "desire, orgasmic capacity and ejaculating capacity" can be intact, even though a man is suffering from E.D. E.D. also does not mean that a man is infertile. The NIH went on to note that millions of men in the United States are affected by E.D. and that this condition can cause mental stress that affects not only the men with the condition, but their partners and entire families as well.

Men and their partners who suffer from E.D. should appreciate that E.D. is not necessarily an "all-or-nothing" phenomenon. For example, E.D. can occur in varying degrees—ranging from complete E.D., whereby a man can never achieve an erection sufficient for intercourse, to an inability to achieve a satisfactory erection intermittently. In other words, sometimes a man may achieve a semi-rigid erection, but the erection is not rigid enough to achieve penetration. Lastly, some men with E.D. have morning erections, but a morning erection is not synonymous with being able to achieve and maintain an erection for sexual activity. Simply stated, then, male erectile dysfunction is now defined as the inability to achieve and/or maintain an erection satisfactory for sexual intercourse.

What is the prevalence of E.D.? We discussed this in detail in Chapter 1, but to review: The National Institutes of Health Consensus Statement, issued just a few years ago, puts the number of men in the United States who suffer from E.D. at ten to twenty million. If men with episodic erectile dysfunction are included, the number then jumps to thirty million. The prevalence of E.D. increases with age; for example, the NIH Consensus Conference stated that E.D. occurs in 5 percent of men aged forty but that 15 percent to 25 percent of men have E.D. at age sixty-five years and older. In the Massachusetts Male Aging Study, 52 percent of the men reported some degree of E.D.; the prevalence rate climbed to 67 percent at seventy years of age. In fact, the prevalence rate may approach a rate of 75 percent in men eighty years of age. As more and more men seek help for E.D., now that an effective oral drug therapy such as Viagra is available, we are likely to see these prevalence numbers climb even higher.

Why Does Male Erectile Dysfunction (E.D.) Occur?

Overall, there are two broad classifications of the causes of E.D.: One is organic, and the second is psychological. It is likely that the majority of patients have an organic etiology, or cause, but psychological factors may also be present, even when there is an underlying organic cause. The most commonly diagnosed causes of E.D. are listed in Table 2, as follows on page 10.

What Are the Risk Factors for Development of Male Erectile Dysfunction?

The purpose of this section is to review some of the key studies that have sought to determine the major risk factors for development of E.D. Many of the risk factors for E.D. are tied in to the organic causes of E.D., listed in Table 2. For example, smoking is a risk factor that leads to acceleration of atherosclerosis, or vascular disease. Vascular disease is, then, an organic cause of E.D., so that smoking can be considered a risk factor because it leads to the development of the organic cause.

Chronic Diseases

Many men in the United States suffer from some type of chronic illness that can cause E.D. To begin, let's take a look at common cardiovascular diseases, such as hypertension, atherosclerosis, and diabetes.

Hypertension: High blood pressure, or hypertension, is an insidious, often ominous disease. Today, the American Heart Association estimates

Table 2

CAUSES OF E.D.

Vascular Diseases
- atherosclerosis
- smoking
- diabetes
- high levels of total cholesterol and LDL cholesterol
- low levels of HDL cholesterol
- hypertension
- combinations of the above
- vascular surgery
- heart disease
- venous leak (a condition in which veins don't collapse fully during erection; therefore, blood drains from the penis)

Neurogenic Disorders
- neuropathies, including diabetic neuropathy
- spinal cord injury
- prostatectomy
- multiple sclerosis
- cerebrovascular accident (stroke)

Endocrine Abnormalities
- hypogonadism (reduced testosterone levels)
- pituitary tumor
- hypo- or hyperthyroidism

Renal failure and dialysis

Psychogenic
- anxiety
- depression
- troubled relationships

Structural Abnormalities
- Peyronie's disease
- priapism

Various Medications
- (Please see Table 5 on page 22, but be sure to consult your physician for specific information.)

that approximately one in four American adults in the U.S. have this disease; of these, about half are men.

Although the disease of hypertension is well known, many people still remain undiagnosed and untreated. Why?—Because hypertension is a silent disease; *i.e.*, there are no symptoms in approximately 90 percent of patients. Regrettably, in fact, sometimes the first sign of high blood pressure is a heart attack or a stroke. Due to the lack of overt symptoms, many men who have E.D. do not realize that they may be hypertensive and that it is this vascular disorder—hypertensive disease— that is causing their E.D., and not a problem that is simply in their heads!

Experts today estimate that about 15 percent of men who are hypertensive experience complete erectile dysfunction at some time. So how does a disease without symptoms manage to inflict such damage and cause E.D.?

The first step in understanding how a vascular disease such as hypertension causes E.D. is to understand and appreciate that the penis is a vascular organ (Figure 3). An adequate amount of blood must enter the penis in order to achieve an erection, and the blood must remain there to maintain an erection. Now, picture your heart as a pump, and the veins and arteries as a network of pipelines. When your blood pressure is elevated, or higher than normal, the pump (your heart) must work harder to keep the blood flowing adequately to the main organs. The more pressure on the pipelines, the more likely they are to undergo de-

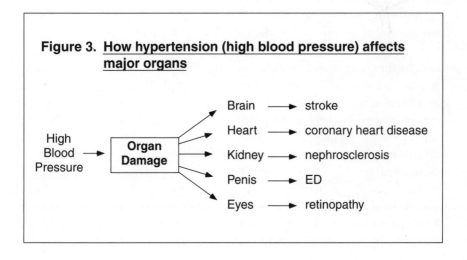

Figure 3. How hypertension (high blood pressure) affects major organs

High Blood Pressure → Organ Damage →

Brain → stroke

Heart → coronary heart disease

Kidney → nephrosclerosis

Penis → ED

Eyes → retinopathy

generative changes and damage. This damage can limit blood flow through the arteries leading to the penis. In this setting, E.D. can occur.

Atherosclerosis: By now, most of us are all too familiar with the litany of reasons why we should stay physically fit and consume a low-fat diet. The culprit we are trying to control is cholesterol, and the reason is that too much dietary cholesterol can lead to a buildup of fatty deposits in the arteries (Figure 4). The main culprit is LDL, or low-density lipoprotein cholesterol, often known as the "bad cholesterol." Conversely, high levels of HDL, or high-density lipoprotein cholesterol (also called the "good cholesterol"), seem to protect us against atherosclerosis.

When does the disease process of atherosclerosis begin? And how do you know whether or not it is contributing to E.D.?

As we discussed, atherosclerosis involves the buildup of fatty deposits in the arteries. The term *atherosclerosis* is derived from the Greek *athera* (gruel) and *sclerosis* (hardening). At the outset, the fatty buildup in the arteries starts out as a thin streak, or plaque, inside the lining of the artery. Later, a "patch" forms, referred to as an *atherosclerotic plaque*. These lumpy plaques can line the arteries, thereby obstructing an adequate blood flow supply through the arteries to key organs. In fact, the plaques can block blood flow altogether, which sometimes occurs in a coronary artery, and a heart attack occurs. Obstructed blood flow in a cerebral or brain artery, on the other hand, can result in a stroke.

Atherosclerosis also limits blood flow through the arteries that lead to the penis. In fact, even atherosclerosis in its very early stages can result in impeding proper function of the arterial tree, thereby reducing its overall ability to supply an adequate flow of blood to the penis.

In order to examine the relationship between E.D. and arterial function further, a group of medical investigators posed this question: Is impotence an arterial disorder? The findings of their study, "Is impotence an arterial disorder? A study of arterial risk factors in 440 impotent men," was published in 1985 in the prestigious British medical journal, *Lancet*. The investigators determined the presence and distribution of four main arterial risk factors: diabetes, smoking, hypercholesterolemia (or elevated cholesterol levels), and hypertension. Overall, 440 men averaging forty-seven years of age participated in the study. An index called the PBPI (penile blood-pressure index, or penile-brachial pressure index) was measured using a special blood pressure cuff. This index compares the blood pressure in the penis to that in the arm. Normally, the ratio is about 0.9

Figure 4. <u>A view inside a coronary artery</u>

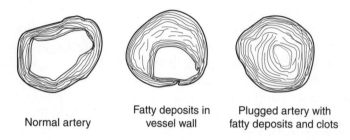

Normal artery   Fatty deposits in vessel wall   Plugged artery with fatty deposits and clots

The open artery on the left is relatively clear of fatty deposits. The middle illustration shows fatty deposits accumulating in the coronary artery; the illustration on the far right shows a nearly clogged, or occluded, artery.

or higher. It takes a pressure-head of about 80 mm Hg in order to achieve an erection. In men with E.D. due to vascular disease, the PBPI is reduced, and a value of less than 0.75 suggests vascular E.D. In some men in this study, the blood vessels going to the penis were also visualized, or examined, by angiography. In this test, a special dye is injected into the blood vessels so it can be visualized during x-ray. This procedure allows the physician to see any narrowing of a blood vessel due to atherosclerosis. In this study, 53 percent of patients who had organic impotence had evidence of such narrowing in their arteries. Overall, the vascular risk factors of smoking, diabetes, and high total serum cholesterol were more common in the impotent men than in the general male population. Diabetes alone, in fact, was associated with a low PBPI (less than 0.9). Whenever two or more of the four vascular risk factors were present, the PBPI was lower. Finally, the frequency of organic E.D. was 100 percent in men with three or four of the vascular risk factors. So again, the same vascular risk factors associated with atherosclerosis in the heart and elsewhere often add up to vascular E.D. Clinicians now know that today atherosclerosic disease is the cause of half or more of E.D. cases in men over fifty years of age. Finally, results of several studies have suggested that low levels of the good cholesterol (HDL) are associated with E.D., whereas high levels of HDL cholesterol seem to protect against E.D. This same pattern is present with atherosclerosis in the coronary arteries; LDL cholesterol makes it worse, and HDL makes it better.

Like hypertension, atherosclerosis also is an insidious disease process. If you see your physician for treatment for E.D., he or she will be able to determine whether or not you need to be evaluated for this condition.

Angina: Simply stated, angina pectoris is nature's warning sign of coronary artery disease. Overall, approximately 7,200,000 U.S. adults have angina today. Of these, nearly three million are men.

One of the earliest and most accurate descriptions of this condition was prepared by the noted British physician William Heberden, who presented a memorable lecture to the Royal College of Physicians of London in 1768. Four years later, in 1772, his work, entitled "Some Account of a Disorder of the Breast," was published. His classic description of anginal pain follows:

> But there is a disorder of the breast marked with strong and peculiar symptoms, considerable for the kind of danger belonging to it, and not extremely rare, which deserves to be mentioned more at length. The seat of it, and sense of strangling, and anxiety with which it is attended, may make it not improperly be called angina pectoris.
>
> Those who are afflicted with it are seized while they are walking (more especially if it be uphill, and soon after eating) with a painful and most disagreeable sensation in the breast, which seems as if it would extinguish life if it were to increase or to continue; but the moment they stand still, all this uneasiness vanishes.

Angina is very easy to understand if we utilize a simple analogy. If you write more checks against your bank account than you have funds available, you create an imbalance; the supply of cash in your bank account cannot meet the demands—the checks come into the bank for collection and your account ends up overdrawn. Of course, if you have sufficient funds available, there isn't any problem.

So, too, is it for the heart. When the myocardium, or heart muscle, pumps sufficient, oxygen-rich blood through the coronary arteries to meet the heart's demands, angina does not occur. Still, this does not mean that some degree of artherosclerosis is not present, since most adults have traces of fatty deposits in their arteries; but overall, the heart is still able to pump sufficient amounts of blood through the coronary arteries to avoid anginal pain. When there is an imbalance in this black-

and-white formula—in other words, when myocardial (heart muscle) oxygen demands exceed myocardial oxygen supply—anginal pain and/ or a heart attack may occur.

The pain of angina pectoris stems from the disease process just described: atherosclerosis. Patients with angina need to discuss sexual activity with their physician. If you and your doctor determine that Viagra is appropriate therapy for you because you also suffer from E.D., then your doctor will provide you with a prescription for the drug. Please be sure to discuss all medications that you are taking with your doctor before you initiate therapy with Viagra. This is especially important in patients with angina, because many of these patients also take nitrates to relieve anginal pain, and taking nitrates is a contraindication to using Viagra. (Please see the heading, "Contraindications to Taking Viagra," in Chapter 7 for more information.)

Clearly, many risk factors for E.D. are the same as those for heart disease; namely, hypertension, total and LDL (bad) elevated cholesterol, decreased HDL (good) cholesterol, atherosclerosis, etc. Abnormalities and stenoses (narrowing) of the penile arterial system may be present in many patients who have coronary heart disease. In one study, for example, E.D. was present in two-thirds of patients who had heart attacks. Another recent study showed that patients with multivessel coronary artery disease were more likely to experience E.D. than if only one coronary vessel was narrow. Thus, patients with vasculogenic impotence should have their cardiovascular risk factors checked and controlled. Again, keep in mind that the penis is a vascular organ. Risk factors that affect the vascular tree affect the *entire* vascular tree.

SEX AFTER A HEART ATTACK

Sexual dysfunction, including loss of libido, and E.D. may be present in heart attack patients. However, this does not mean that post-heart attack sexual dysfunction is permanent. Psychogenic factors may play a significant role in men following a heart attack. For example, many of Dr. Kloner's patients fear that the activity and exertion involved in sexual relations will precipitate another heart attack. This same fear may also be expressed by the partner. As always, you should consult your physician if you have any questions. (Please see "Can Having Sex Cause a Heart Attack?" in Chapter 7.)

Diabetes: Regrettably, the number of adults in the United States who have diabetes is growing. Today, the American Diabetes Association estimates that approximately 15.9 million adults in the U.S. have diabetes; of these, about 7.5 million are men.

Briefly, diabetes is a disorder of metabolism, the body's regulating process in which foods are broken down into their constituent chemicals and rebuilt into new substances, or broken down and transformed into other chemicals that may be eliminated from the body or reused.

But in diabetes, the body's ability to utilize carbohydrates—which is a key part of the metabolic process—is impaired. The result? Sugars accumulate in the blood in excess and ultimately are eliminated in the urine. One hormone—insulin—which is produced by the pancreas, is key in the metabolism of sugars. In diabetes, the amount of insulin produced by the pancreas is insufficient or the body develops resistance to insulin; thus, the body cannot adequately metabolize carbohydrates.

Two types of diabetes are known: Type 1 diabetes, formerly known as juvenile diabetes, and Type 2, or noninsulin dependent diabetes mellitus (NIDDM).

What is the link between diabetes and E.D.? Actually, medical researchers have known for some time that diabetes is among the more common physical causes of E.D. Clinicians have since learned that diabetes and E.D. so often go hand-in-hand that in approximately 12 percent of men, E.D. is the first overt sign of diabetes.

In one study, for example, 365 men with Type 1 diabetes, in which the onset of diabetes occurred prior to the age of thirty, were followed serially. Overall, 20 percent reported a history of erectile dysfunction. Their average age was 37.6 years. The frequency of E.D. increased from 1.1 percent in patients twenty-one to thirty years of age to 47.1 percent in men over forty-three years of age. Men with diabetes for thirty-five years or more were 7.2 times more likely to report E.D. than men with diabetes of ten to fourteen years' duration. The investigators concluded that a high frequency of E.D. occurs in young diabetics and postulated that better control of glucose levels might help.

If you have diabetes, or any of the warning signs of diabetes (see Table 3), you need to see a physician for diagnosis and a proper medical treatment strategy. Diet and exercise both play important roles in keeping diabetes under control. Although it is true that many men with diabetes experience occasional episodes of E.D., it is also true that over half the men with diabetes who were given Viagra for E.D. responded favorably

Table 3

WHAT ARE THE WARNING SIGNS OF DIABETES?

___

There are numerous symptoms associated with diabetes:
- chronic hunger
- chronic thirst
- frequent urination
- skin infections (boils, carbuncles—painful, pus-bearing inflammations of tissue beneath the skin)
- vaginal itching
- visual disturbances
- weakness, malaise
- weight loss*

* Weight loss is particularly noteworthy when it occurs despite a good appetite and adequate food intake.

___

to the drug. Today, thanks to Viagra, many men with diabetes have an opportunity to restore erectile function to normal or near-normal.

At this point, it's worth repeating that the penis is a vascular organ. Thus, factors that adversely affect the blood vessels and cause damage and alterations in the function of these blood vessels, or cause frank atherosclerotic narrowing of these vessels, may also affect the penis and cause E.D.

Neurogenic E.D.

Other organic problems that can cause E.D. are nerve damage or spinal cord injury, as well as other traumatic nerve damage due to surgery and/ or disorders of the nervous system that may inhibit erection.

Spinal cord injury: Men with a wide range of spinal cord injuries frequently suffer from E.D. In fact, the results of one study published in 1960 revealed that half of 529 men with spinal cord injuries in either the upper or lower motor neuron lesions—and only half who attempted intercourse—were able to achieve erections that allowed for successful sexual intercourse.

Structural Abnormalities

Lastly, an organic problem such as Peyronie's disease, for example, which is an abnormal fibrosis of the corpus cavernosum (the spongy erectile tissue), can cause E.D. Priapism, on the other hand, is an abnormal erection that occurs without sexual arousal in the presence of certain diseases such as sickle cell anemia. Priapism can result in eventual damage to erectile tissue.

Surgeries: Two types of pelvic surgery in particular—transurethral resection of the prostate (TURP) and radical prostatectomy (a procedure performed to treat prostate cancer) often cause E.D. in men. Today, thanks to the introduction of Viagra, many of these men are now receiving an acceptable form of treatment for their E.D., and many are responding very favorably to the drug.

Other Organic Diseases, Disorders, and Risk Factors for E.D.

In addition to such common cardiovascular disorders as hypertension, angina, atherosclerosis, and diabetes, a wide range of other diseases and disorders can also cause E.D. These include kidney disease—most notably, chronic renal failure (RF), liver failure, multiple sclerosis, and Alzheimer's disease. Too, several endocrine disorders, such as hypo- and hyperthyroidism, hypogonadism and hyperprolactinemia commonly cause E.D. Interestingly enough, E.D. is also found in approximately 30 percent of men with chronic obstructive pulmonary (lung) disease. Finally, the Massachusetts Male Aging Study reported that E.D. was also associated with untreated ulcer, untreated allergies—even untreated arthritis.

Depression: One could easily ask: Does E.D. cause depression, or does depression cause E.D.? Again, findings from the Massachusetts Male Aging Study uncovered this: A whopping 90 percent of men who were considered severely depressed reported moderate or complete E.D. In addition, men who were assessed as suffering from moderate depression, as well as men who claimed only a minimal degree of depression, experienced moderate or complete E.D. nearly 60 percent and 28 percent of the time, respectively.

Depression stems from two causes: endogenous, meaning coming from within, and exogenous, meaning coming from something outside. For

Table 4

ARE YOU DEPRESSED? KNOW THESE WARNING SIGNS

- feelings of anxiety
- loss of appetite
- sleeplessness (insomnia)
- weight loss
- loss of interest in things you usually enjoy
- feelings of sadness
- suicidal thoughts
- low self-esteem
- poor self-image
- consistent feelings of anger

example, it's reasonable to understand why any man might experience a bout of depression if he loses his job, has a seriously ill child, and so on. On the other hand, endogenous depression occurs when you experience feelings of sadness or a loss of interest in your hobbies with no tangible reason to explain the falling mood (see Table 4).

Highly respected author William Styron, for example, seemed to have it all: marriage, children, a beautiful home in Connecticut, and a very successful career as a best-selling author and screenplay writer (his novel, *Sophie's Choice* was also made into an award-winning film). Yet several years ago, Styron's mood simply sank; that is, his mood altered so severely that he was no longer able to write. Ultimately, he became so depressed that he felt overwhelmed by the simple task of brushing his teeth in the morning. This type of depression, of course, is considered very severe; Styron was hospitalized for several months, recovered from the depression, and received subsequent medication to treat the depression. Shortly after his recovery from depression, Styron wrote *Darkness Visible*, which recaps, in exquisite detail, his odyssey to the brink and back again. Mike Wallace, the famed CBS co-host of the television program "60 Minutes," has also told his story of depression. He received appropriate drug therapy and continues to lead a full and productive life at seventy-six years of age.*

---

*The authors wish to make clear that these are descriptions of men who have experienced clinical depression and received medical treatment for the depression. These cases are cited to illustrate how common depression is, and that it can strike anyone. There is no intent to suggest or imply that either of these men ever reported being diagnosed or treated for E.D.

Regardless of the type of depression you may have, if you are also suffering from E.D., it is possible that these two conditions may be exacerbating each other. In fact, results of one study revealed that both expression *and* suppression of anger were associated with a greater likelihood of moderate and complete E.D. In addition, men who tended to be more dominant and controlling of their environment and trying to influence others experienced E.D. To find out more about how effective Viagra is in combatting E.D. in depressed men, please see Chapter 7.

Alcoholism: Today, the pitfalls of excessive drinking and alcohol abuse are well known; acloholism is now recognized as a treatable disease. So, it's no surprise to learn that ingesting more than minimal quantities of alcoholic beverages, especially coupled with aging, often results in E.D.

Heavy drinking—three or four drinks per day or more—can ultimately lead to neuropathy, a form of nerve damage that can inhibit the nerve signals needed for erection. If you consult your physician about E.D., he or she, in the course of taking and/or reviewing your medical history, will likely ask you about your drinking patterns. Be sure to be totally honest; after all, no physician or prescription can help you effectively and appropriately if you are not candid with your doctor.

Cigarette smoking: Do you remember a public health campaign from the past:

> If you smoke cigarettes, stop.
> If you don't smoke, don't start.

That says it all, really. Is there anyone, anywhere, today who can say anything positive about cigarette smoking? Added to all the other health risks are results of clinical studies that showed cigarette smoking as major risk factor for E.D. in patients who had either heart disease or high blood pressure. Overall, 56 percent in the group of men evaluated, of current smokers who had treated heart disease, were impotent, compared to 21 percent of current nonsmokers. Patients who were taking various heart disease and high blood pressure medications were much more likely to experience E.D. if they also smoked. The message here is very clear: If you have heart disease or high blood pressure and you are also taking medicines for these conditions, *and* you smoke, then you are much more likely to have E.D. than if you don't smoke—or stop smoking today.

Medications: There are a whole host of medications, both prescription and over-the-counter, that can trigger E.D. Please look at Table 5 to check whether you are taking any of these medications. If you are, and you also suffer from E.D., please let your doctor know what medications you take regularly so he or she can guide you and modify or change your treatment, if necessary. If that doesn't work—meaning that normal or near-normal erectile function isn't restored—then your physician may prescribe Viagra for you.

Psychological origins: Is E.D. all in your head? The truth is, it sometimes can be, although we now know that it is just as likely to be due to the presence of one or more of the organic diseases just discussed, as well as some medications you may be taking or some of your "bad habits" (such as cigarette smoking or using recreational drugs). Certainly anxiety, depression, and emotional difficulties are also associated with E.D. Sometimes these psychological factors are transient and due to specific situations, such as loss of a job, difficulties in a relationship, serious illness in the family, and so on.

Again, if you are experiencing E.D., consult your physician. After a frank conversation and a review of your medical history, he or she will be able to determine with you what the next step should be. If you don't smoke, for example, and organic diseases don't seem to be the root of E.D., then your health care professional may recommend some counseling, along with a prescription for Viagra. Over time, it is very likely that you will be able to resume satisfactory sexual intercourse.

Aging: Most of us would readily agree that aging has its pitfalls; hopefully, with proper exercise and diet, many of us can lead healthy and productive lives well into our seventies and eighties. Still, as we age, we do need to pay careful attention to our health, and staying healthy includes maintaining sexual health. Many women today are leading the march toward a healthy sexual life, into and beyond menopause. Now, their partners can follow suit: Men who suffer from E.D. should consult their physicians for evaluation and treatment with Viagra, if indicated, just as women today see their gynecologists for estrogen patches, vaginal lubricants, and so forth.

Remember, as we discussed in Chapter 1, the Massachusetts Male Aging Study found that age is a risk factor for E.D. Complete E.D. was reported in 5.1 percent of forty-year-old men and increased to 15 per-

Table 5

SELECTED LIST OF MEDICATIONS ASSOCIATED WITH
ERECTILE DYSFUNCTION

Please consult your physician before making any changes in your
medications. Other medications besides those listed here may also
cause E.D.

Antihypertensives
- Diuretics (especially thiazide diuretics)
- Beta-blockers
- Centrally acting agents

Other Cardiovascular Drugs
- Clofibrate
- Gemfibrizol
- Digoxin

H$_2$ Antagonists (for ulcers)

Non-steroidal Anti-inflammatory Drugs (for pain, arthritis)

Antidepressants
- Selective Serotonin Reuptake Inhibitors (SSRIs)
- Tricyclic antidepressants

Hormones
- Corticosteroids
- Estrogens
- Antiandrogens

Other Substances and Drugs
- Alcohol
- Cancer chemotherapeutic agents
- Cocaine
- Marijuana
- Narcotics
- Opiates
- Tobacco

cent for seventy-year-old men. Moderate E.D. increased from 17 percent
in forty-year-old men to 34 percent in seventy-year-old men. Age re-
mained an important variable for the development of E.D. even after
correcting for other variables.

Figure 5. The many faces of erectile dysfunction

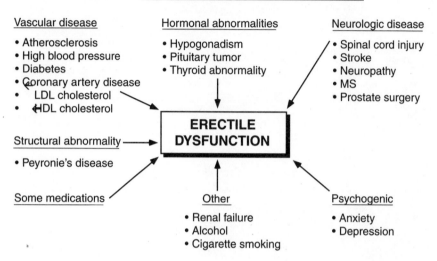

As discussed earlier, after adjusting for age, certain common diseases were significantly associated with E.D.; namely, diabetes, heart disease, and hypertension.

So what does all of this mean for you and your partner? Clearly there are some risk factors for E.D., such as cigarette smoking, that you can eliminate, and there are other risk factors you can modify successfully. For example, if you have a high total cholesterol level, or LDL cholesterol, you can diet and/or take medication to reduce your cholesterol level (see Figure 5). If, on the other hand, you have low HDL cholesterol, you can increase your HDL cholesterol level by increasing your level of exercise and/or taking medication. Lastly, if you are a heavy drinker, you should cut back.

There are other factors, however, that we cannot control; aging is one. If you need surgery for prostate cancer, that's another risk factor for E.D., but clearly appropriate management of the cancer is the goal.

Fortunately, the birth of Viagra has led to another medical disorder coming out of the closet quickly: E.D. Now, men and their partners are not only more willing to discuss this problem openly, but more and more couples are seeking effective medical treatment. Now that you know what male E.D. is, please see your physician if you need help. Both you and your partner will benefit, possibly for many years to come.

3

The Almighty Erection
Here's How It Works

"Birds do it, bees do it, even educated fleas do it"
—COLE PORTER, 1928

Actually, though, this line from Cole Porter's 1928 song is not quite true. Such creatures procreate, yes, but some species of animals don't "do it," at least as we've come to know "doing it"—that is, having sexual intercourse. In fact, only vertebrates "do it"—animals such as dogs, cats, elephants, hippos, lions, tigers, bears, monkeys, baboons, gorillas, and man. The act of "doing it," or having successful sexual intercourse, at least at a bare minimum, requires the male species to have an erect penis sufficient enough to achieve penetration.

In man, how does penile erection occur? Certainly by the time a young man is in his teens, he can rattle off the answer: "I feel horny, I get an erection." We asked a couple of young men in college, and both replied along those lines: "I see a gorgeous girl, that's it! I get an erection!" "I've been dating a fantastic girl for three months—it's difficult for me to be around her, out at night, and *not* get an erection!"

But that's only telling us how these young men respond to visual sexual stimulation; it's *not* telling us how and why the erection occurs.

To understand more about what actually takes place physically to trigger an erection, we need to revisit "Anatomy and Physiology 101." Here goes!

25

What is an Erection?

An erection is defined as rigidity of the phallus that enables sexual activity to occur. Penile erection is dependent upon a complex interaction among hormones, nerves, blood vessels, and muscle tissue.

Pathways to Erections

Overall, there are three major pathways to erection: nocturnal, reflexogenic, and psychogenic.

Nocturnal erections: While you sleep you pass through various stages of sleep, one of which is called the "rapid eye movement"—or REM—period because of the rapid eye movements that are known to occur during this stage. REM sleep normally occurs two to three times a night and typically lasts from ten to twenty minutes each time. Dreams can occur during the REM stage of sleep and so, too, do erections, but the exact neurologic pathway causing the nocturnal erections remains unknown. Because dream sleep often occurs just before awakening, men frequently experience early morning erections.

Reflexogenic erections: Direct stimulation of the penis—that is, touch (reflexogenic)—may create an erection via a lower spinal cord pathway that returns the activating signal directly back to the penis (see Figure 6). In fact, even if the spinal cord is disconnected from the brain by an upper spinal cord injury, this mechanism still works. This is referred to as "sarcogenic sex" because a man with a spinal cord injury is not aware that he has this erection, nor does he experience pleasurable feelings due to the disconnection to the brain.

Psychogenic erections: A centrally mediated or psychogenic erection is initiated in the sexual centers located within the brain. These centers are activated by various erotic stimuli, including sights, sounds, smell, taste, and thoughts. The sexual centers then stimulate the penis through either the spinal cord or extra spinal pathways.

During typical sexual activity multiple mechanisms come into play; for example, arousal comes into play through erotic stimulation in areas within the brain. This mechanism is at least partially dependent upon

Figure 6. This illustrates the human nervous system demonstrating the potential neural pathways controlling erection. Stimuli that reach the brain through the senses will stimulate an erection through the upper spinal cord (T11 through L2) and the hypogastric nerves. However, direct stimulation of the penis, transmitted through the dorsal nerve of the penis, will stimulate an erection through a reflex arc located in the lower spinal cord (S2 through S3).

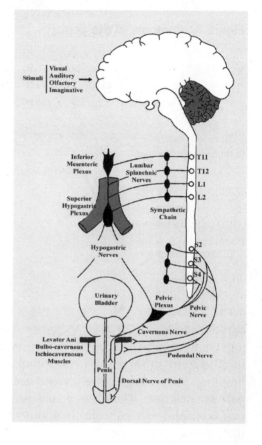

stimulation of the brain by male hormones. Direct tactile stimulation (touch) of the phallus reinforces this central mechanism to create full erection. Unfortunately, the aging process sometimes adversely effects the penis's ability to respond to these neural stimuli. Thus, an older man may no longer be able to achieve a full erection in response to just erotic stimuli; he may require additional active stimulation to achieve erections satisfactory for sexual intercourse.

Anatomy of an Erection

The penis: The human penis is made up of three cylindrical bodies: the corpus spongiosum (spongy body), which contains the urethra and includes the glans penis, or head of the penis, and the paired corpora cavernosa, or erectile bodies (see Figure 7). The corpus spongiosum cylinder engorges or fills with blood when an erection occurs, but this cylinder does not provide any significant rigidity to the erection. The paired

Figure 7. <u>Anatomy of the penis</u>

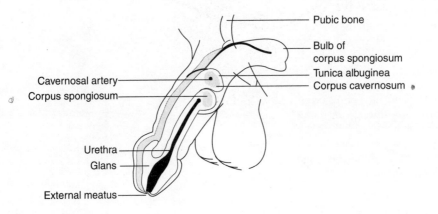

Pubic bone

Bulb of
corpus spongiosum

Tunica albuginea

Corpus cavernosum

Cavernosal artery

Corpus spongiosum

Urethra

Glans

External meatus

corpora cavernosa, or erectile bodies (two bodies that function as one unit), are actually responsible for the erection. They provide the structural support to the erect penis. Similar to a beam extending out of a building, the erectile bodies extend deep into the body in order to support the erection. Thus, the actual penile length includes the amount that is visible externally and an additional length that extends deep into the pelvis.

Now, think of a banana. The outer covering, or peel, is analogous to the tough elastic outer covering of the paired erectile bodies and is called the tunica albuginea, which encloses each of the corpora cavernosa. The cavernosal tissue—analogous to the banana pulp—is made up of fine-walled empty spaces, similar to a common sponge. Unlike a sponge at your kitchen sink, however, the sinusoidal tissue in the penis fills with blood rather than water. Then, like a sponge that fills with water, this sinusoidal tissue expands as it fills up with blood. The sinusoidal tissue is composed of vascular epithelial cells that line the cavernosal empty spaces and a special type of muscle called smooth muscle.

Blood reaches the penis via arteries within the center of the erectile bodies called the cavernosal arteries (see Figure 8). The blood drains from the penis through three sets of veins: the superficial, the intermediate, and the deep dorsal veins. The latter—the deep dorsal veins—drain

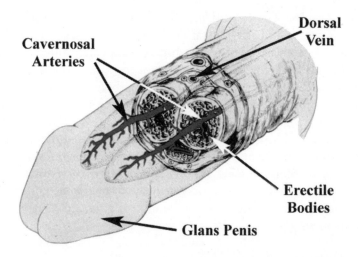

Figure 8. This illustration of the human penis depicts the paired erectile bodies located in the shaft of the penis. The glans penis, or head of the penis, is connected to the urethra located below the erectile bodies. Each erectile body has a central, or cavernosal, artery which supplies the blood needed for an erection. The dorsal vein is located outside the erectile bodies and drains blood away from the penis and back into the body.

blood from the corpora cavernosa and the corpus spongisum, or head of the penis.

Nerves: Various nerves are responsible for transmitting signals back to the brain in order to experience tactile (touch) sensation and for transmitting signals to the penis to either stimulate or inhibit an erection. Nerves that transmit external stimuli signals to the spinal cord and brain are called "afferent nerves." Nerves that originate in the brain and spinal cord and send signals to the penis are called "efferent nerves." The dorsal nerve of the penis runs the entire length of the penis; it is an afferent nerve. The cavernous nerves originate deep in the pelvis and run between the prostate and rectum, to enter the erectile bodies at the base of the penis. Cavernous nerves are the main efferent nerves; they are responsible for stimulating an erection. But the cavernous nerves are also mixed nerves; as such, they contain both inhibitory and excitatory nerve fibers. Because the cavernous nerves are located near the prostate and rectum, they are vulnerable to injury during both prostate and rectal surgery.

Smooth Muscles: The key element necessary for the production of an erection is smooth muscle relaxation. That's right, relaxation. This is the opposite to what you might have intuitively expected, since most physiological processes require an active event to initiate them instead of a passive event. In a manner of speaking, the body is almost always actively preventing an erection by the contraction of the smooth muscles that line the vascular spaces within the erectile bodies. In fact, development of an erection is almost a passive event, since the only thing required is the *relaxation* of these very same muscles. This relaxation results in dilating the blood vessels, thus, blood flows into the penis. Smooth muscles are not consciously or voluntarily controlled by the brain. Smooth muscles within arteries are examples of muscles that work without your having to think about them.

Skeletal muscles: The base of the erectile bodies is surrounded by skeletal muscles. The muscles, called the bulbospongiosus and ischiocavernosus muscles, are able to contract around the base of the erectile bodies. The contraction of these muscles greatly increases the pressure within the erectile bodies during erection, thereby producing extremely rigid erections. With contraction of these muscles, the pressure inside the erectile bodies can even exceed normal blood pressure. These muscles are under conscious or voluntary control, similar to muscles in your arms and legs. Ultimately, these muscles automatically contract as part of the ejaculatory process.

The Erectile Mechanism

An erection of the human penis is a vascular event that involves nerves, smooth muscle, and vascular endothelium (the cells that line the blood vessels and sinusoidal spaces within the erectile bodies). In a normal flaccid, or nonerect state, the smooth muscles are contracted around the arteries and sinusoidal tissue. This muscular contraction limits blood flow into the penis, preventing the penis from filling up with blood. At this point, the sinusoidal tissue is like a dry sponge. In the flaccid state, the blood flows directly through the sinusoids into the veins exiting the erectile bodies and, ultimately, the dorsal vein (see Figure 9a and 9b). In order to achieve an erection, the blood flow into the penis has to increase and the blood must be trapped within the penis.

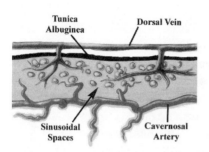

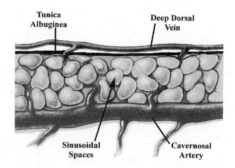

Figure 9a. This illustration represents a cross-section of a single erectile body within the penis when the penis is not erect. The cavernosal artery is located in the center of the erectile body and carries the blood into the penis. Without an erection, the sinusoidal spaces are empty and there is free efflux of blood through the outer covering of the erectile body, tunica albuginea, into the dorsal vein.

Figure 9b. This illustration depicts what happens inside the erectile bodies during an erection. The central, or cavernosal artery, dilates and the sinusoidal spaces fill with blood because of smooth muscle relaxation. As the sinusoidal spaces expand, the veins draining blood out of the erectile bodies are compressed underneath the tunica albuginea, which prevents venous leakage.

Steps to an erection: First, neural stimulation of smooth muscle relaxation within the walls of the penile arteries and sinusoidal tissue occurs. The relaxation of the smooth muscles of these arteries and sinusoids is dependent upon release of certain chemicals following nerve stimulation. One of these chemicals, called nitric oxide (NO) is crucial for relaxation of smooth muscle in the penile blood vessels (see Figure 10). Smooth muscle relaxation reduces the resistance to blood flowing into the penis, and sinusoidal tissue sucks up blood like a sponge. As the sinusoidal tissue expands within the tough elastic tunica albuginea (the banana peel), the veins become trapped and compressed under the inner surface of the peel of the erectile bodies. Thus, the inflow of blood into the penis exceeds the outflow, and the penis is able to fill with blood. In the initial stages of an erection, this produces engorgement (tumescence). The ultimate size and shape of an erection is determined by the limited elasticity of the peel, or tunica albuginea. Disorders of the tunica albuginea that affect its elasticity can disfigure the shape of an erection. Peyronie's disease, for example, which is a type of "arthritis" of the penis, often affects the size and shape of an erection.

Once the penis has filled with blood, called tumescence, a mechanism to occlude or block venous outflow of blood must function in order to maintain the erection. The occlusion mechanism of these veins

Figure 10. Steps to an erection

The male body relies on two chemicals to trigger, achieve, and maintain an erection satisfactory for sexual intercourse. Here's how the chemical pathways work:

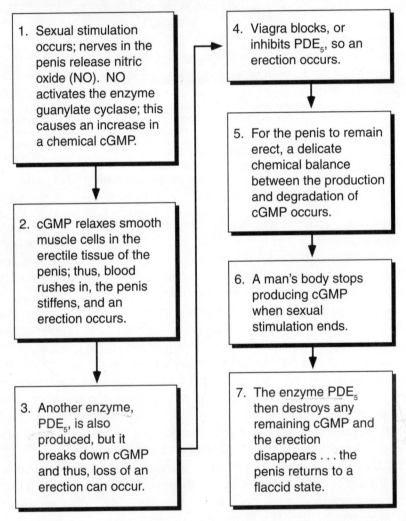

1. Sexual stimulation occurs; nerves in the penis release nitric oxide (NO). NO activates the enzyme guanylate cyclase; this causes an increase in a chemical cGMP.

2. cGMP relaxes smooth muscle cells in the erectile tissue of the penis; thus, blood rushes in, the penis stiffens, and an erection occurs.

3. Another enzyme, PDE$_5$, is also produced, but it breaks down cGMP and thus, loss of an erection can occur.

4. Viagra blocks, or inhibits PDE$_5$, so an erection occurs.

5. For the penis to remain erect, a delicate chemical balance between the production and degradation of cGMP occurs.

6. A man's body stops producing cGMP when sexual stimulation ends.

7. The enzyme PDE$_5$ then destroys any remaining cGMP and the erection disappears . . . the penis returns to a flaccid state.

occurs by the passive compression of the veins under the tunica albuginea (refer to Figure 9). Failure of this mechanism results in a "venous leak"—in other words, it becomes difficult to maintain an erection without continuous maximal stimulation of blood flow into the penis.

To help understand this better, just think of filling a pail of water with a garden hose. If the hose isn't damaged, a large amount of water can flow through it and it is quite easy to fill the pail. But if the hose is clogged, similar to arterial occlusive (blocking) disease, or you cannot turn on the faucet—in other words, a neurological disease is present— then it becomes difficult or even impossible to fill the pail. Now, assume that someone punches a small hole in the bottom of the pail, say with an ice pick. That's a small venous leak! It becomes even more difficult to fill the pail and keep it full. But if you have an undamaged garden hose, it shouldn't be a problem. If, however, someone cuts off the entire bottom of the pail, then a large venous leak occurs—in other words, it becomes impossible to fill the pail, no matter how much water flows through your garden hose. Clearly, the vascular events involved in producing human erection require a delicate balance between arterial inflow and venous outflow that favors the arteries. These vascular events are dependent upon three events—smooth muscle relaxation, passive venous occlusion, and skeletal muscle contraction—in order to produce maximal penile rigidity sufficient for sexual relations. Very little blood flows into the erectile bodies when the penis is fully erect. If a full erection lasts too long—say, greater than three hours—damage may occur to the erectile tissue due to a lack of adequate oxygenation. This disorder is called priapism, named after a Greek god of fertility, Priapus, who had a permanent erection.

Upon orgasm and ejaculation, inhibitory efferent nerves release chemicals that cause contraction of smooth muscles within the arterial walls and sinusoidal trabecula. Smooth muscle contraction decreases blood flow to the erectile bodies, and the veins open up to drain the sinusoidal spaces. When blood drains away from the penis back into your body, loss of erection, or detumescence, occurs.

What About Male Hormones?

Virtually everyone has heard of testosterone, the king of the male hormones, but what does it do and what role does it play in erections? You may be surprised to learn that although male hormones are an important aspect of normal sexual function in man, they are not critical for sexual function. The main male hormone in the bloodstream is testosterone, which is produced by Leydig cells located in the testes.

After the Leydig cells produce testosterone, this hormone circulates in the bloodstream and exerts its effect upon target organs and tissues such as the brain, bones, muscles, and penis by diffusing into the cells. Once inside the cell, testosterone may act unchanged or be metabolized into other active hormones. A breakdown product of testosterone is dihydrotestosterone (DHT); it is much more potent than testosterone. Certain sites in the body need DHT rather than testosterone—for example, the prostate as well as the hair follicles. Drugs are now available that prevent the conversion of testosterone into DHT, and these drugs are now used to treat prostatic disorders and male pattern baldness.

Testosterone production in the testes is controlled by a hormone, luteinizing hormone (LH), which is produced by the pituitary gland located in the brain. The pituitary gland controls both testosterone and sperm production within the testes. In general, sperm production is much more vulnerable to outside disruption than testicular hormone production. Therefore, many insults that adversely affect testicular sperm production have little or no effect upon the amount of testosterone in the blood. The pituitary gland, in turn, is controlled by the hypothalamus, which is a tiny part of the brain located just above the pituitary gland. The hypothalamus secretes a hormone, gonadotropin-releasing hormone (GnRH), which stimulates the pituitary gland to secrete LH. The hypothalamus is the "mission control center" for male hormone production, continuously incorporating signals from various parts of the body in order to meet the body's myriad demands. Testosterone itself is involved in its own regulation by exerting feedback inhibition upon the secretion of both GnRH and LH; in other words, testosterone functions like a thermostat in your home. When testosterone levels are low, the brain produces more LH in order to stimulate testosterone production in the testes. Conversely, a high level of testosterone lets the brain know there is an adequate amount of male hormone available, and the signaling to the testes is turned off until the level of testosterone in the blood starts to fall. Estrogen, a female hormone, is also present in men, albeit at very low levels. The primary source of estrogen in men is conversion of testosterone to estrogen by fat cells in the body. As such, obesity can result in an excess of female hormones in a man.

Interestingly enough, the exact role of testosterone in male sexual function is not clear. It seems that it is limited to maintenance of sexual drive or libido in the adult. Testosterone is also necessary for the development of the penis during fetal development: a lack of testosterone during this time period results in a very small penis, called microphallus. The rising testosterone level associated with puberty, on the other hand, is responsible for growth of the phallus during adolescence. The adult has considerably higher levels of testosterone, but penile growth ceases following puberty, even when testosterone is given as a supplement. Studies show that men without testosterone can still achieve erections. In other words, testosterone is not critically necessary for the erectile mechanism. Measurement of nocturnal erections demonstrate that the erections of men with low testosterone levels are less strong and occur less frequently during the night, but are still within the normal range. However, recent laboratory studies have shown that testosterone does enhance the function of the nerves within the penis, suggesting that although it is not absolutely necessary, testosterone does play a contributory role to the overall erectile mechanism.

Prolactin: Another hormone produced by the pituitary gland that has no known function in the male but can interfere with sexual and reproductive function is prolactin. In women, prolactin is secreted by the pituitary gland during and after pregnancy to stimulate milk production by the breasts. Elevation of prolactin levels in the blood inhibits the secretion of GnRH by the hypothalamus which, in turn, lowers testosterone levels by the lack of LH signaling to the testes. This same mechanism also occurs in women, which explains why women do not often become pregnant while breastfeeding.

Chemicals: Over the last decade, researchers have learned a great deal about the mechanism of penile smooth muscle relaxation, which has led to many advances in the diagnosis and treatment of E.D. For example, we know that during sexual stimulation a substance called nitric oxide (NO) is released in the spongy erectile tissue of the penis, called the corpus cavernosum. NO activates an enzyme called guanylate cyclase, which causes an increase in the substance cyclic guanosine monophosphate (cGMP). cGMP is a key factor in causing an erection because it relaxes the smooth muscle cells in the erectile tissue of the penis, thereby allowing blood to rush into the spongy tissue. At this point, the penis stiffens and a man has an erection. Men with E.D. often lack sufficient cGMP. Viagra *increases* the levels of cGMP in erectile tissues by inhibiting another enzyme, phosphodiesterase type 5, or PDE_5, which breaks down cGMP and can result in the loss of an erection. This enzyme, PDE_5, is found almost exclusively in the penis. Thus, administering substances that increase the amount of either NO or cGMP within the penis can potentiate an erection. One way to accomplish this is to prevent the degradation, or breakdown, of cGMP (refer to Figure 10).

For example, Viagra (sildenafil citrate), is a phosphodiesterase inhibitor that is specific for the phosphodiesterase type 5 (PDE_5) present in the penis (see Figure 11). Viagra prevents the breakdown of the active form of cGMP and amplifies any signal sent to the penis.

As in most designs of nature—or even those created by man—there are backup systems: in case one fails, the other takes over. This is also true for the erectile mechanism of the penis. In addition to the NO system incorporating cGMP as the second messenger (see Figure 11), there is another system that incorporates a second messenger, called cyclic adenosine monophosphate (cAMP). To date, most of the medications that have been used in the management of erectile dysfunction prior to the advent of Viagra utilized the cAMP pathway to produce an erection. Prostaglandin E_1, for example, stimulates the production of cAMP directly, whereas the drug papaverine is a nonspecific phosphodiesterase inhibitor that inhibits the enzyme that degrades cAMP.

What Can Go Wrong with an Erection?

Overall, there are four physiological mechanisms by which an erection can go awry. The first and least common is hormonal; the second is neurologic, which is one of the more common mechanisms, particularly if you count psychogenic erectile dysfunction as neurologic. The remaining two mechanisms are vasculogenic.

Hormonal Pitfalls

The hypothalamic-pituitary-gonadal axis is responsible for maintaining normal levels of testosterone in the bloodstream. The most common cause of a low testosterone level is testicular dysfunction, which may occur at any point in a man's life but is more common in elderly men.

Figure 11. How VIAGRA works to help you achieve and maintain an erection

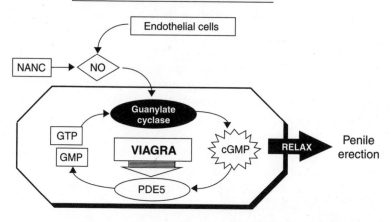

NO is released from neurons and endothelial cells (lining the arteries), increasing the amount of smooth muscle cGMP. Increased levels of cGMP are involved in smooth muscle relaxation; this, in turn, leads to penile erection. Next, cGMP is converted back to GMP by PDE$_5$. Viagra is a highly selective inhibitor of PDE$_5$ and prevents the breakdown of cGMP; thus, premature loss of erection does not occur.

NO = nitric oxide
NANC = nonadrenergic-noncholinergic neurons
GTP = guanosine triphosphate

GMP = guanosine monophase
cGMP = cyclic guanosine monophase
PDE5 = phosphodiesterase type 5

Adapted with permission from Ignarro, L.J., et al. *J Pharmacol Exp Ther.* 1981; 281: 739–749

Although testosterone has little direct effect upon the penis, the effects of a low testosterone level are manifested by reduction in libido, also known as sex drive. A much less common, but also a very important cause of a low testosterone level is a pituitary tumor. These brain tumors are benign and do not metastasize, but they can cause a great deal of damage to the brain if left untreated. The tumor's main adverse effect upon erectile function is mediated by its reduction of sex drive.

Neurologic Damage

Damage to the neural pathways that normally stimulate an erection can prevent the signals from reaching the penis. Spinal cord injury, for example, is the most prevalent cause of neurologic E.D. However, nerve damage may be even more insidious than that. Diabetes mellitus, as has been discussed in Chapter 2, is a common metabolic disorder that can often be associated with subtle nerve damage. In fact, many men with diabetes have E.D. as their *first* symptom of this disorder. Diabetes mellitus can also have an adverse effect upon the small arterial blood vessels, which can interfere with the normal erectile mechanism. In diabetic patients with E.D., it is often difficult to ascertain whether the primary pathology is in the nerves or the blood vessels. Another, less common neurological disorder that causes E.D. is multiple sclerosis (MS). MS is a chronic, degenerative disorder of the nerves that has an insidious onset. Patients may have mild to moderate symptoms for years prior to the establishment of an actual diagnosis of MS.

Pelvic surgery, such as removal of the prostate for prostate cancer, can also damage the nerves and result in E.D. Fortunately, increased knowledge of the neural anatomy supplying the penis has allowed for the development of surgical techniques that can now spare the nerves responsible for an erection while still removing the entire prostate.

Vascular Diseases

In Chapter 2, we discussed how several types of vascular disorders can adversely affect erections. One is arterial occlusive disease; the most common cause of this is atherosclerosis, or hardening of the arteries. This condition is often a result of elevated LDL cholesterol, cigarette smoking, and hypertension. In addition, trauma and surgery can cause a blockage in the arteries that carry blood to the penis. The other vascular cause of E.D. is veno-occlusive dysfunction. As mentioned previously, the venous occlusive mechanism is a passive one. Any abnormality within the penis that prevents expansion of the sinusoids within the erectile bodies will result in continuous leakage of blood out of the penis. Thus, the wear and tear of age alone may induce E.D. through fatty deposits in the walls of the sinusoidal tissue, which can adversely affect its ability to expand and compress the veins that carry blood out of the penis. Trauma to the penis, particularly fracture of the erect penis, can result in the deposition of scar tissue within the erectile bodies and ultimately interfere with normal erectile function.

Psychological Interference

In some ways psychogenic E.D. is a separate category, but its mechanism can also be classified within other categories. Since it originates from the brain, psychogenic erectile dysfunction can also be considered neurologic. However, the most common cause of psychogenic E.D. is "performance anxiety," which produces a venous leak-like picture. An anxious person secretes catecholamines from the adrenal gland; it's called the "fight or flight" reaction. This response is a very important survival reflex that allows the body to mobilize its forces for a life-important moment—for example, if you are suddenly awakened during the night because you hear someone breaking into your house. In this reaction, catecholamines secreted by the adrenal glands stimulate the heart to beat faster and stronger, and the blood pressure rises. All of these events sound like they may be good for an erection, since an erection is dependent upon blood flow. But catecholamines are also a strong stimulant of smooth muscle contraction, which is the exact *opposite* of what you need to achieve an erection. In fact, catecholamine-like substances are released at the time of ejaculation to make an erection subside, a process known as detumescence. The smooth muscle contraction interferes more with venous occlusion than with the arterial inflow, which is why patients with psychogenic E.D. appear to have veno-occlusive dysfunction upon routine testing.

E.D.: What To Do Next

If you are experiencing consistent difficulty in achieving an erection sufficient for satisfactory sexual intercourse, you and your partner should talk it over and determine whether or not both of you think it's time to consult a physician. To determine whether or not you have erectile dysfunction, why not begin by taking a look at Chapter 4 of this book: it's designed to help you assess what you should do . . . and when.

4

You Think (or Know) You're Impotent
What Should You Do?

Paul and Sarah couldn't believe it. For a while, Paul assumed he was just exhausted, and both he and his wife, Sarah, recognized that nothing kills an erection like plain old fatigue. Just over a year ago, Paul had decided to retire. He'd held a terrific position as a senior executive with his company for thirty-two years; now, he and Sarah determined it was their turn to "kick back" and have some fun.

By early spring 1998, both he and Sarah were very excited, anticipating a relaxing new life together. They were also in the throes of preparing for three major life-event changes: his retirement; the youngest of their three children, Jeremy, was graduating from college and heading off to medical school, and their only daughter, Erica, was getting married. By early July 1998, however, everything had settled down—settled down quite a bit, in fact. Sarah and Paul had to acknowledge that since the spring, they simply had not been able to enjoy satisfactory sexual intercourse because of Paul's inability to sustain an erection.

Was Paul impotent? Sarah wondered. And if so, why? Worse yet, why now? Sarah brought up the subject with Paul one evening after dinner, as they discussed planning a late-summer ten-day cruise. Sure, fatigue had been an issue in the past—often, for both of them—but the transition to retirement had been an easy adjustment. Both Sarah and Paul thought their sexual activity would increase, not decline! Paul assured

Sarah that it was certainly not for lack of desire; he still cherished Sarah and looked forward to a happy and enjoyable retirement with her. After a heart-to-heart talk, they decided to seek medical help. From that point on, the rest, as they say, is history.

The couple were evaluated by Paul's physician, including a physical checkup for Paul. His blood pressure was too high, and he was given appropriate medication. At that time, he was also given a prescription for Viagra to treat his E.D. Both Sarah and Paul today report that all's well—and retirement couldn't be better!

The purpose of this chapter is to help you assess whether you have E.D. and what your next step should be.

1. Ask Yourself: Do I Have E.D.?

One of the easiest ways to determine whether or not you have E.D. is simply to review the medical definition of E.D., and then ask yourself whether or not your sexual performance falls within these boundaries:

> Erectile dysfunction is a medical condition in which there is an inability on the part of the male to achieve an erect penis as part of the overall multifaceted process of male sexual function. This includes the ability of the male to **attain** and **maintain** erection of the penis sufficient to permit satisfactory sexual intercourse.

If you answer yes to one or both parts of this description, then you have E.D. Still, it's also important to remember that there are *grades* of E.D. For example, if you are able to achieve an adequate erection 95 percent to 99 percent of the time and only have difficulty 1 percent to 5 percent of the time—and it doesn't particularly bother you or your partner—then the degree of erectile dysfunction may not be serious enough for you to want to seek help. On the other hand, if that 1 percent to 5 percent of the time that you do have problems achieving an erection is so psychologically troublesome for you—that is, you feel horribly depressed and/or anxious as a result—then perhaps you should get medical attention. Certainly, those men who *usually* fail to achieve an erection with sexual activity should consider a medical consultation. Ultimately, of course, the decision of whether or not you should go to your physician and discuss the problem of erectile dysfunction is up to you—and your partner. The fact that there is now an oral pill that is effective in many men with E.D. means that there is a high likelihood that, if you seek help with E.D., you will, in fact, resolve your E.D.

2. It Takes Two, So Keep Your Partner in the Loop

Often, it's the partner who has a heightened awareness of E.D.; this person may be more "tuned in" to how often the E.D. occurs. Because so many men become both anxious and depressed about E.D., their partners may detect certain behavioral patterns that encourage them to avoid sexual encounters: for example, retiring to bed very late, excessive drinking, or even initiating an argument before bedtime. Your partner may be the one who notices this pattern of behavior and calls it to your attention. If you think that you have minimal or no problem with E.D., but your partner disagrees, it's worth discussing the issue with your mate. Then, consider obtaining help from a health care professional. Remember, "it takes two," and the satisfaction of your partner is an important element in the equation of when to obtain professional help for E.D.

Is Viagra a "Quick-Fix?"

The advent of Viagra may lead to a tendency for men to want the "quick-fix"—to take Viagra without an evaluation. We know, for example, that some men are already trying to convince their primary care providers to write a prescription for Viagra without so much as even coming in for a consultation! In our opinion, this approach is a mistake. First, E.D. often indicates that there are risk factors for other diseases present, and one or more of these may warrant medical treatment. Your physician needs to evaluate the presence of these risk factors, and he or she must select a course of treatment appropriate for you. Proper medical therapy now can possibly reduce life-threatening medical events, such as a heart attack or stroke, in the future.

Also, as we discussed in Chapter 2, a whole host of medical conditions—high blood pressure, diabetes, neurologic disorders, and so forth—can cause E.D., as can some of the treatments for these maladies. However, when you see your health care professional for a consultation, he or she will then review your entire medical status with you. If one or more of the medications you are taking seems to be the underlying cause of your

E.D., then your physician may decide to change your medication alto-gether, and thereby eliminate the E.D. you are experiencing, or may pre-scribe Viagra. An adequate medical evaluation allows you and your health care provider the opportunity to determine whether or not your E.D. is psychogenic; if so, this can be treated with appropriate psychological therapy.

3. Whom Do I Go to See?

The answer to this question is really up to you and your partner. In our managed-care climate, your health care plan may dictate with whom you can consult. For example, many managed-care plans mandate that you consult your primary care physician first. The primary care physi-cian often serves as the "gate-keeper," and he or she can determine whether or not a referral to a specialist such as a urologist, cardiologist, etc., is necessary. If your E.D. is due to taking certain high blood pres-sure medicines, for example, or you are experiencing transient psycho-logical difficulty (such as performance anxiety, anxiety and/or depression related to divorce, conflict with a business partner, and so forth), then your primary care physician may feel it's appropriate to manage your E.D. If, on the other hand, your E.D. is possibly due to a more complex medical or surgical condition, such as post-prostate surgery, Peyronie's disease, or hypogonadism due to testicular failure, then the primary care physician may refer you to a specialist.

In other managed-care plans, you may be able to consult a specialist, such as a urologist, directly. If this is the case—and you feel more com-fortable seeing a urologist—then by all means do so. In general, urolo-gists are well trained in evaluating men for E.D., and they still tend to have the most experience in diagnosis and selecting treatments, although this is now changing rapidly due to the introduction of Viagra.

Clearly, the availability of Viagra is affecting the physician-prescrib-ing landscape. Now, more and more physicians, physician's assistants, and nurse practitioners are quickly becoming versed in their knowledge of E.D.: causes, risk factors, and treatment options.

If you suspect you have E.D. and want to seek help, review your health care plan to see what alternatives are available. Ask your provider, for example, whether there are certain physicians in the plan who specialize in impotence/E.D.; ask for a list of those professionals. If your health care plan does not permit this, then see your primary care physician as your first step. Your physician may decide to evaluate and treat you at that time, or you may be referred to a specialist, depending upon the cause, severity, and what your physician sees as the prognosis of your condition.

4. Preparing for the Patient (or Patient/Partner) Interview

Okay—so now you and your partner have made it to the doctor's office. Both of you should heave a sigh of relief because the worst part of the problem—recognizing E.D. and showing a shared willingness to deal with it—is over!

Now, in order to help your health care provider help both of you, it's useful to know what types of questions he or she is likely to ask when you come in for the initial office visit. If you are a regular patient, your doctor will talk with you for a few minutes to see how you are feeling overall, review any medications that you may be taking, and so on. If you are a new patient, the doctor will begin with a thorough medical and sexual health history, then conduct a physical examination with basic laboratory tests. Either way, the doctor ultimately has to determine the answers to the following questions:

- Do you truly have E.D.?
- If so, how severe is it?
- How often is it a problem?
- Is it due to an organic cause?
- Is it due to a psychogenic cause?
- Is it due to a cause that can be corrected?
- Are there other risk factors for E.D. present that should be treated?

To help evaluate your E.D. most effectively, some physicians will provide you with a patient questionnaire; your candid answers will help your health care professional determine the next steps. This questionnaire may be given to you either before you see the doctor for the first time, or after the first visit.

Among other things, the questionnaire will ask you whether or not your partner is interested in your receiving treatment, and, if so, whether or not you are amenable to having your partner included in discussions with you and your physician. Next, your doctor needs to know about your ability to have an erection and the frequency of your erections. If possible, he or she will likely ask you to rate the degree of rigidity, in hardness, of your erection on a scale. For example, a scale of one to ten might be used, where ten is a normal erection that you might have experienced in your twenties and one is an inability to have an erection at all. Several different scales are currently being used by different physicians. A simple but effective scale was published within the last two years in the highly respected *British Journal of Urology* (see Figure 12). You may be asked to "rate" your erections according to this scale.

Do you achieve an erection, and then lose it? Your doctor needs to know this, as well as whether you can achieve an erection with masturbation and whether you have normal erections in the morning or upon awakening during the night. This is an important question because it may help the physician to determine whether your E.D. is due to psychogenic or organic causes. Men with psychogenic E.D., for instance, usually have normal nocturnal and early morning erections. An exception to this is severe depression. If you have normal erections at night and in the early morning hours, it suggests that key nerve pathways and circulatory systems are intact. Also, a history of sudden-onset E.D. may suggest a psychogenic cause. For example, a traumatic event such as

Figure 12. <u>Grading your erection: a sample scale</u>

1 Increase in size of penis but no hardness

2 Increase in size and slight increase in hardness (rigidity), but insufficient for sexual intercourse

3 Increase in hardness (rigidity) sufficient for sexual intercourse, but not fully rigid

4 Fully rigid erection

Reproduced with permission from Boolell, M., Gepi-Attee, S., Gingell, J.C., Allen, M.J. Sildenafil, a novel effective oral therapy for male E.D. *Br J Urol.* 78 (1996) 257–261.

Table 6

IS IT ERECTILE DYSFUNCTION?
START WITH THE AT-HOME CHECKLIST

YES	NO	
❑	❑	You routinely cannot achieve an erect penis, and it bothers you and your partner.
❑	❑	You consistently cannot attain and maintain erection of the penis sufficient to permit satisfactory sexual intercourse.
❑	❑	You and/or your partner feel that there is some degree of erectile dysfunction present, possibly in a sufficient degree to warrant a medical consultation.

If you answered yes to even one of these questions, you should consider a medical consultation.

loss of a loved one, loss of a job, or other personal tragedy may result in an abrupt onset of psychogenic E.D. Organic E.D., on the other hand, is usually associated with a gradual onset.

Besides questions about erections, the questionnaire may also ask you about sexual desire, or libido. Again, a scale may be provided for you to rate your sexual desire. Your partner may be asked to rate his or her sexual desire on the same scale, too. Frequency of sexual encounters—or attempted sexual encounters—are also evaluated, as well as your ability to achieve orgasm (climax). Whether or not you experience premature ejaculation or painful ejaculation is also an item for review.

Finally, the questionnaire asks about certain risk factors that are relevant for both E.D. and cardiovascular risk. For example, are you a smoker? Do you drink alcohol—and, if so, how much? Do you have high blood pressure, diabetes, cholesterol abnormalities, or a history of heart disease?

If you are taking any medications, the questionnaire will cover that, too. Before you visit your doctor, write down a list of all of the medications you take, their doses, and the frequency and duration of your taking them. This list should include *all* over-the-counter remedies, including aspirin, cough/cold tablets, and so on. If you take organic nitrates, or in the past have taken organic nitrates such as nitroglycerin, *be sure* to discuss this with your physician. Prior surgeries, or any prior treatments

Table 7

PREPARING FOR THE OFFICE VISIT

Think about your overall health—if you've had any problems recently, from headaches to indigestion, a dizzy spell, any sleeplessness, and so on. Be prepared to inform your physician.

Do you have a history of heart disease?

Are you taking any medications? (Note frequency and doses.)
  • Prescription drugs (including any and all forms of nitrates)
  • Over-the-counter medications such as:
    aspirin
    cough/cold tablets
    muscle relaxants
    pain relievers
    laxatives
    antacids

• **Think about your sexual history in detail.**
    • How often do you have satisfactory sexual intercourse?
    • Are your erections hard?
    • Do you get an erection, and then lose it?
    • Can you have an erection to masturbate?
    • Are you still interested in sex?
    • Do you have early morning erections (*i.e.*, when you awaken)?

---

for E.D., need to be addressed as well. Of course, there are many other questions that your doctor may ask you, but these are among the most common ones. Reviewing these questions and what your answers will be may help you, your partner, and your physician move the evaluation forward (see Tables 6 and 7). To learn more about a medical workup and evaluation for E.D., simply move on to Chapter 5!

5

The Male Erectile Dysfunction (MED) Checkup

Don't worry. It's highly *unlikely* that you'll be the first patient your doctor sees with E.D. As the baby boomers—that's us—cross the "50-divide," we visit our physicians more often. We do this not just for treatments, but to stay healthy—and maintaining sexual health is a priority for us, too. Keep in mind, however, that different physicians have different approaches to the management of E.D., so in this chapter we'll first discuss the reasons why your physician may use a particular approach. Also, we're going to cover the questions your physician will ask you to determine the type of sexual disorder present and how to manage it best for you. Lastly, we'll take a look at the reasons why routine and more sophisticated laboratory studies and diagnostic tests are performed.

For most physicians, the first step in the evaluation of a man with E.D. is to rule out any serious underlying medical disorders, gain a rough idea as to the cause of the condition, and educate both the man and his partner regarding current treatment options. Do note: Most physicians like to see the partner, too.

Clinical experience shows that the exact cause of E.D. has little impact upon the choice of therapy, and here's why. Factors that carry much more weight in selecting treatment are the man and his partner's preconceived notions regarding treatment, the ease of use, and the lack of significant risk. Moreover, there are only a limited number of medically significant diseases that need to be evaluated carefully for E.D., and this can almost always be accomplished with minimal laboratory testing, such as blood tests. In other words, there's no need to brace yourself for a gamut of time-consuming, expensive, and/or painful diagnostic procedures.

Traditionally, physicians have performed a complete evaluation on every patient who complained of E.D. Sometimes, this involved extensive testing, which was indeed both costly and time consuming. The complete evaluation generally consisted of a thorough history and physical examination by a qualified specialist, laboratory testing (blood work), assessment of nocturnal erections, and vascular testing. All of these tests cost several thousands of dollars, and yet it was still possible that the exact diagnosis of E.D. could not be established upon the completion of the evaluation. What was often discovered was that by just talking to and examining a patient with E.D., an experienced physician could arrive at the same diagnosis in most men—without all the procedures. Furthermore, we now also know that the exact diagnosis as to the cause or etiology of E.D. does not always affect the choice of therapy. Still, there are a few situations in which it can be important to know the exact cause of the E.D. before initiating treatment. For example, the most common scenario is that of a young man in whom one might suspect a curable cause of E.D., such as elimination of cigarette smoking or a medication; in another case, a man may be involved in litigation and need to document the exact etiology. Finally, there are some men who just want to know for certain whether or not the cause of their E.D. is physical or psychological. But keep in mind that all of these settings are the exception—rather than the rule—and therefore, most men with E.D. do not require a complete laboratory and psychological evaluation.

Goal-Directed Therapy

Over the last decade, following the development of multiple effective nonsurgical therapies, a more tailored approach to the management of men with E.D. has taken hold. This approach, called goal-directed or goal-oriented therapy, takes into account the patient's wishes, desires, and goals of therapy. Fortunately, most clinicians today recognize that this approach is appropriate for the vast majority of men with E.D. who are seen today.

What is goal-directed therapy? Specifically, it is composed of a history and physical examination, minimal laboratory testing, and patient education. Patient education is a *crucial* component of this approach since it is so important for the patient and his partner to understand the pros and cons of all of the available treatment options *before* making an informed decision regarding the management. Using this approach, a doctor will only order a test if it is appropriate to the patient's choice of therapy. Among other things, this approach produces a significant cost savings and allows for more rapid initiation of therapy, since no matter how long a man has had E.D., once he has taken the giant step forward of discussing his problem with a physician, he generally wants to start treatment as soon as possible.

Causes of E.D. and Therapeutic Options

We have already presented the causes of E.D. at length in this book, but these factors also play an integral role in goal-oriented therapy, so we need to re-visit them here.

The primary causes of E.D. are physical and/or psychological, or organic and psychogenic, respectively (see Table 8). Typically, causes can be distinguished based on a man's history alone. As outlined in Chapter 2, your physician will consider various physical etiologies, including hormonal abnormalities, vascular disturbances, and neurologic disorders. Few men have a "pure" E.D. problem. In fact, almost all men with a physical cause of E.D. also have a psychogenic component. The stress— and distress—E.D. causes can emotionally wear many men down. It is not uncommon for a man to convert a partial problem of E.D. into a complete one because he worries whether or not he can achieve a successful erection next time. Before you know it, a man with occasional E.D. finds himself in the grip of complete E.D. due to performance anxiety.

Treatment options for E.D. consist of counseling or sex therapy, oral medications (pills), drugs that are administered directly into the penis by either injection or insertion into the urethra, hormonal therapy, vacuum erection devices, penile prosthetic surgery, and vascular surgery.

We generally classify treatment options as either specific or nonspecific (see Table 9). Specific therapies are those that are only effective if the patient has a specific etiology; for example, administering testosterone to a man with a low testosterone level. Testosterone therapy, on the other hand, is not effective for men with normal testosterone levels. Likewise, sex therapy can only be fully effective if there is a significant psychogenic component. True, sex therapy for a man with significant vascular

Table 8

E.D.: IS THE CAUSE ORGANIC OR PSYCHOGENIC?

	Organic	*Psychogenic*
Duration	Longstanding	Recent onset
Onset	Gradual	Sudden
Quality	Constant	Intermittent
Erection at orgasm	Flaccid	Full or unable to orgasm
Nocturnal erections	Absent	Present

Table 9

SPECIFIC AND NONSPECIFIC THERAPIES FOR E.D.

SPECIFIC THERAPIES

Etiology (cause)	*Therapy*
Psychogenic	Sex therapy
Hormonal	Hormonal therapy
Neurogenic	Injection therapy
Arterial occlusive	Vascular surgery

NONSPECIFIC THERAPIES

Oral medications
Vacuum erection devices
Injection therapy
Penile implants (prostheses)

disease may help him adjust to the problem, but it certainly will not cure his E.D.

Finally, some treatment options can be used both as specific therapies and as nonspecific therapies. (Viagra is a nonspecific therapy because it works in patients with organic and/or psychogenic causes.) Injection therapy, for one, is a specific therapy for neurogenic E.D. The injection of a vasodilating medication directly into the erectile bodies replaces the normal signal that would be transmitted by the nerves. However, unlike many other specific therapies, injection therapy, at high doses, can effectively treat E.D. in the vast majority of men, no matter what the cause. Minimal evaluation is needed for those patients requesting nonspecific therapy modalities, since the actual cause of E.D. is unimportant. In contrast, a patient who desires corrective vascular surgery requires a much more extensive evaluation to determine the exact etiology and to determine whether or not surgery is an appropriate treatment option.

The History Tells Your Story

The patient history is the most important part of any evaluation. In fact, in 1993 the NIH Consensus Panel stated that the appropriate assessment of men with E.D. should include the following:

- a medical history
- a sexual history
- a physical exam

Why? During a medical history, the physician asks many questions that are quite personal in an effort to determine the exact problem and gain some insight into the root of the problem. First, he or she tries to determine what type of problem is troubling the patient, since many different problems can present, or be described as, E.D. Specifically, though, E.D. is primarily a problem of obtaining or maintaining sufficient penile rigidity to engage in sexual intercourse. Many men also have problems with orgasm, which they can confuse with the problem of E.D. Similarly, many men experience bouts of premature ejaculation and anorgasmia, and they confuse this with E.D. as well. In fact, premature ejaculation is actually a relative term since it is defined as the inability to delay orgasm long enough to satisfy both sexual partners. Premature ejaculation may be confused with E.D. because the erection normally subsides with orgasm and, therefore, the loss of erection may be thought of as a manifestation of E.D. Conversely, many men with E.D. develop premature ejaculation because of the need for intensive penile stimulation to avoid the loss of the erection during sexual relations. In anorgasmia, or retarded ejaculation, the opposite occurs. There are very few known physical causes of anorgasmia, other than certain antidepressant medications and head trauma. As such, patients with retarded ejaculation are often referred for sexual therapy to treat the disorder. Another disorder commonly confused with E.D. is Peyronie's disease. Peyronie's disease is a connective tissue disorder of the penis, or "arthritis" of the penis, that is characterized by painful, bent erections. Patients with Peyronie's disease are prone to E.D. However, the E.D. associated with Peyronie's disease is managed quite differently; that is, in approximately 20 percent of patients, the disease resolves itself. Other patients with Peyronie's disease require surgery to straighten the penis or to insert an implant. Thus, it is very important to identify Peyronie's disease early and to make certain that a specialist is involved in its management. The key questions used to determine whether or not Peyronie's disease is present is for the physician to ask about a new onset of penile curvature with erections, pain in the penis associated with an erection, or a palpable area of hardness ("knot") within the penis.

Describing Your E.D.: Once it has been established that the primary problem is E.D., the nature and course of the E.D. need to be defined further. The first set of questions asked by the physician are:

- How long has the problem been present?
- Was the onset gradual or sudden?
- Is the E.D. constant or intermittent?

These questions are used to differentiate between organic and psychogenic E.D.

In general, long-standing E.D. of gradual onset and constant degree are consistent with a physical problem. However, a sudden onset of E.D. following pelvic surgery, for example, or the institution of new medical therapy for high blood pressure is also strongly suggestive of an organic etiology. Conversely, as has been previously mentioned, sudden onset of E.D. following a death of a spouse or job loss is more suggestive of a psychogenic etiology. Your physician may use a professionally developed scale, called the International Index of Erectile Function (IIEF) to assist him or her in his evaluation of your E.D. (see Table 10b at the end of the chapter). You will be asked to complete or fill out the questions on the scale as completely and honestly as possible. An abbreviated form of this scale can also be used (see Table 10a).

Your Level of Erectile Function: The next set of questions assesses your current level of erectile function. The questions are:

- How good an erection do you achieve with sexual stimulation?
- How full are your early morning erections?
- How rigid is your penis at time of orgasm?

Table 10a

SEXUAL HEALTH INVENTORY FOR MEN — IIEF-5:
AN ABBREVIATED SCALE

Patient's name

Date of evaluation

Patient Instructions

Sexual health is an important part of an individual's overall physical and emotional well-being. Erectile dysfunction also known as impotence, is one type of very common sexual complaint. There are many different treatment options for E.D. This questionnaire is designed to help you and your physician identify if you may be experiencing E.D. If you are, you may choose to discuss treatment options with your doctor.

Each question has several possible responses. Circle the number of the response that best describes your own situation. Please be sure that you select one and only one response.

Over the past six months:

1. How do you rate your *confidence* that you could get and keep an erection?

   1   Very low
   2   Low
   3   Moderate
   4   High
   5   Very High

2. When you had erections with sexual stimulation, *how often* were your erections hard enough for penetration (entering your partner)?

   0   No sexual activity
   1   Almost never/never
   2   A few times (much less than half the time)
   3   Sometimes (about half the time)
   4   Most times (much more than half the time)
   5   Almost always/always

3. During sexual intercourse, *how often* were you able to maintain your erection after you had penetrated (entered) your partner?

0   Did not attempt intercourse
1   Almost never/never
2   A few times (much less than half the time)
3   Sometimes (about half the time)
4   Most times (much more than half the time)
5   Almost always/always

4. During sexual intercourse, *how difficult* was it to maintain your erection to completion of intercourse?

0   Did not attempt intercourse
1   Extremely difficult
2   Very difficult
3   Difficult
4   Slightly difficult
5   Not difficult

5. When you attempted sexual intercourse, *how often* was it satisfactory for you?

0   Did not attempt intercourse
1   Almost never/never
2   A few times (much less than half the time)
3   Sometimes (about half the time)
4   Most times (much more than half the time)
5   Almost always/always

Score _____

Add the numbers corresponding to questions 1 to 5. If your score is 21 or less, you may be showing signs of erectile dysfunction and may wish to talk to your doctor.

- Do you have trouble getting an erection?
- Do you have difficulty maintaining an erection?
- Have you undergone any prior testing for E.D., including blood work?
- Have you tried any treatments for E.D., prescribed by a physician or otherwise?

Again, for example, ability to achieve full erections under certain settings but not in others suggests a psychogenic etiology. The presence of full erections during the night or upon awakening with a full bladder is also suggestive of a psychogenic cause. But the questions the doctor asks are not always reliable, since men may report the loss of nocturnal erections but still have them while in deep sleep, and therefore not be aware of them. In working with many E.D. patients, Dr. Jarow has found that the most reliable question is whether or not the penis is erect or flaccid at the time of orgasm. Most men—and many physicians in fact—are unaware that a man can ejaculate without an erection. But almost all men with organic E.D. are aware of this phenomenon, since they have experienced it for themselves. Many men who are unable to climax, since they are not relaxed enough to achieve orgasm, have psychogenic E.D. Performance anxiety often lies at the heart of their E.D. Table 10 outlines how clinicians generally distinguish between organic and psychogenic causes of E.D.

Can You Maintain an Erection? The next set of questions is aimed at determining the type of erection problem that is present. One may be a problem of attaining an erection; the other is difficulty in maintaining it. Experiencing difficulty in attaining an erection is suggestive of either a neurogenic or arteriogenic etiology, whereas difficulty in maintaining an erection is often suggestive of either psychogenic E.D. or veno-occlusive dysfunction. Most men with E.D., however, generally say that they have difficulty both obtaining and maintaining an erection. These questions are important because patients who have difficulty maintaining erections alone can sometimes be successfully managed with the use of constrictive bands at the base of the penis to prevent loss of the erection during sexual relations.

If you have seen other physicians in the past for the treatment of your E.D., you know what tests were done and what treatments were tried. You should be prepared to provide as much information and detail as possible, so your physician does not repeat tests that have already been performed. Occasionally, a doctor will repeat a test if he or she feels the result may have changed since the test was last performed. Knowing the results of previous treatments can assist you and your physician in determining what remaining treatments may work and provide your physician with clues as to the cause of the E.D.

Your doctor or health care provider will also take a complete urologic and medical history to determine potential reversible causes of E.D. Sex drive (libido), past sexual development during puberty, and prior fertility may indicate whether or not there is a hormonal abnormality. A history of trauma to the penis (*i.e.*, buckling during sexual intercourse), trauma to the perineum—that is, bicycle injury and trauma to the pelvis (a pelvic fracture)—may also indicate the cause of E.D.

Neurologic disease or trauma can also be a risk factor for E.D. Spinal cord injury and/or head trauma may lead to problems with orgasm, ejaculation, and erections. Other neurologic disorders that are associated with E.D. include multiple sclerosis, Parkinson's disease, Lou Gehrig's disease (amyotrophic lateral sclerosis), and stroke. Finally, diabetes mellitus is strongly associated with E.D., and the causes can be neurologic, vascular, or both.

Your Vascular Risk Factors: Your physician will also ask you about vascular risk factors in your history. These include high blood pressure, cigarette smoking, diabetes mellitus, hypercholesterolemia (elevated LDL cholesterol), low HDL cholesterol, and the presence of atherosclerotic vascular disease elsewhere in your body. Atherosclerosis is a systemic disease affecting blood vessels throughout the body. Penile arteries are particularly prone to atherosclerosis; as such, E.D. secondary to the presence of vascular disease may actually serve as a harbinger of vascular disease elsewhere in the body. Signs of atherosclerotic vascular disease elsewhere in the body include coronary artery disease (angina or a history of a heart attack), a history of stroke and claudication (pain in the calves while exercising but relieved by rest). The presence of vascular risk factors in your history is a strong indicator that the E.D. is due to physical causes.

Your Drug History: Lastly, your physician will also want to know about your intake of pharmacologic agents, including prescription drugs, over-the-counter medications, and recreational drugs such as marijuana and alcohol. Many medications list E.D. as a potential side effect, and those prescription drugs most likely to cause E.D. are medications used in the treatment of high blood pressure. Antidepressants may also have an adverse effect upon both erectile function and ejaculation. Still, there are very few oral medications that will prevent a normal young man from obtaining an erection, indicating that men who develop E.D. secondary to any of these medications must have underlying problems that have made them vulnerable to E.D. This is particularly true for men with both hypertension and elevated cholesterol levels who probably have underlying vascular disease. It is worthwhile to discontinue medications or switch these medications whenever possible—under a physician's supervision—but keep in mind that you are using these medications to treat a serious medical disorder; no one ever died of E.D., and E.D. is treatable.

And what about alcohol? Actually, there is a very interesting relationship between alcohol and E.D. In light moderation, alcohol can enhance erectile function because it decreases anxiety and releases inhibitions. However, at higher levels alcohol has a very deleterious effect on erectile function. In addition, chronic alcohol abuse results in liver damage, which in turn will produce hormonal imbalances that interfere with sexual function. Chronic alcohol abuse also damages nerves (alcoholic neuropathy), which can also lead to E.D.

The goals of the medical history, then, are to determine the *exact* nature of the sexual complaint, identify risk factors for E.D. that may be reversible or may only serve to identify the underlying cause, and ascertain which diagnostic tests and treatments have been performed, if this is not the first consultation for E.D. With these tasks complete, the next step is the physical exam.

Physical Examination

Even if your physician has seen you on an annual basis for a checkup, he or she is likely to examine you again to check for physical attributes that may provide some insight as to the cause of the E.D. as well as to rule out significant underlying medical pathology. The physical examination will include a measurement of your vital signs (blood pressure, respiratory rate, and so on), a general physical examination, and a specific examination of the male genitourinary system.

- *Vital signs.* Of the vital signs—blood pressure, respiratory rate, pulse, temperature, height, and weight—blood pressure is the most important as related to the complaint of E.D. As mentioned previously, elevated blood pressure is a significant risk factor for vascular disease.

- *Excessive weight.* Obesity is a risk factor for E.D. for three reasons. First, obesity is an independent risk factor for vascular disease. Second, obesity often leads to the development of type 2 diabetes. And third, testosterone is converted into female hormones by fat cells. Obese men often have low blood levels of testosterone.

The general physical examination actually begins the moment you enter your doctor's office, where your general well-being is assessed: How well do you look? Do you move about the office easily? An obvious example of this immediate physical assessment occurs when a spinal cord injury patient enters the office in a wheelchair, in which case the cause of E.D. is immediately clear. Similarly, a patient with significant cardiac or respiratory disease may demonstrate shortness of breath upon moving through the office. More subtle findings are the secondary sex characteristics, which may indicate the presence of a hormonal abnormality. For example, men normally develop temporal balding with age. The absence of this finding may be indicative of a low testosterone level. Sparse facial hair (and pubic hair) may also be indicative of a lifelong low testosterone level. Likewise, having extremely long limbs—eunuchoid appearance—is suggestive of a chromosomal abnormality that results in low testosterone levels for life.

Other aspects of the general physical examination include listening to the heart and lungs as well as palpating the stomach to detect any gross abnormalities of the major organ systems of the body. During this part of the examination, the breast tissue is assessed to ascertain whether there is a hormonal imbalance. Also, a stethoscope is placed on the abdomen to listen for bruits—murmurs that are caused by turbulent blood flow through an atherosclerotically narrowed aorta. Elevated levels of prolactin or the female hormone, estradiol, as well as low testosterone levels may result in enlargement of the male breast (gynecomastia). Finally, assessment of peripheral pulses, particularly those in the feet, will detect the presence of significant vascular disease if they are absent.

Examination of the male genitalia includes assessment of the penis, testes, and prostate. The size and shape of the penis is assessed. The most common cause of loss of penile length is obesity. In addition, the penis becomes smaller with disuse. The penile shaft is palpated very carefully to identify areas of hardness consistent with Peyronie's disease. In men who have not been circumcised, the ability to fully retract the foreskin is checked. The size and consistency of the testes are measured as an indicator of testosterone production. Loss of testicular volume, called testicular atrophy, is an indicator of a low blood level of testosterone. All men with normal-size testes have normal testosterone levels, but the converse is not true. Some men with very small testes still have normal testosterone levels. A digital rectal examination is performed on all men over forty-five years of age as part of routine screening for prostate cancer. A neurologic examination—testing for sensation, strength, and reflexes—may point to a neurologic cause for E.D. Reduced rectal sphincter tone may also suggest a neurologic problem.

Laboratory Studies

Usually, routine screening laboratory studies are conducted on all men who complain of E.D. in order to detect relatively infrequent but significant metabolic and hormonal disorders that are associated with this disorder. Typically, simple blood and urine samples do the trick. A urinalysis and fasting blood sugar are ordered to help the physician detect undiagnosed diabetes mellitus. Clearly, these tests are unnecessary if the patient is already known to have diabetes.

Additional blood tests are conducted to check lipid levels and hormone levels. An elevated blood cholesterol level is a very treatable risk factor for vascular disease. Since vascular disease is one of the more common causes of E.D., it is important to check the blood lipid profile and correct any lipid abnormalities if you have this problem. Finally, endocrine testing should also be performed, and blood levels of testosterone and prolactin are checked. Other endocrine evaluations, such as thyroid tests, may be obtained, too.

Vascular Evaluation

Since vascular abnormalities are the most common cause of physical problems with erections, your doctor will suspect one of two types of vasculogenic E.D.: arterial occlusive disease (insufficient inflow) and veno-occlusive dysfunction (venous leak). In many patients, the history and physical examination provide enough information to establish the diagnosis of vasculogenic E.D. Documentation of penile vascular disease is necessary in only a very small percentage of patients. The main indication is for those patients with suspected arterial occlusive disease who may be potential candidates for vascular surgery, but this represents less than 1 percent of the total population of men with E.D. The second reason to perform a vascular evaluation is to document the cause of the E.D. because of a patient's need to know, or at the request of insurance carriers. Vascular evaluation plays a more prominent role now than in the past when the treatment options for E.D. were quite limited and surgical therapy with insertion of a penile prosthesis was almost the only choice for men with a physical cause of E.D. In contrast, most patients today can now be treated with nonsurgical forms of therapy, making it less important to document a physical or vascular case of E.D.

Duplex ultrasonography is the best test available today to assess the penile blood flow. Duplex ultrasonography is used throughout the body to assess blood flow to a variety of organs, including the heart, brain, and kidneys. Ultrasonography uses sound waves to image internal organs, similar to the concept of sonar used by the Navy to detect submarines. In the absence of radiation, this test is very safe; it is the one used to look at the fetus inside pregnant women. The combination of ultrasound with a Doppler—referred to as "duplex"—allows the physician to detect the vessels inside the erectile bodies and measure the blood flow within these blood vessels. The Doppler is similar to that used by meteorologists to see storms; similarly, your physician detects and measures movement within your body. This test is performed following the injection of a vasodilating drug into the penis, in order to measure the blood flow in the vessel responsible for an erection while an erection is being stimulated. Although duplex ultrasonography is not 100 percent accurate, it is currently the best noninvasive test to assess penile blood flow.

Arteriography is an invasive test that is performed in patients who have abnormal duplex ultrasound study, in order to obtain a "road map" of the penile vasculature prior to performing vascular surgery. This study requires the introduction of a catheter into the arterial system of the body in order to inject contrast and take pictures of the penile arteries. Because there are risks of injury to the arteries associated with this test, arteriography is only performed upon select patients who are found to be candidates for surgical repair of vasculogenic E.D., based upon results of the duplex ultrasound studies.

Nocturnal Erection Assessment

Measurement of nocturnal erections is an objective method to determine whether a man has organic or pychogenic E.D. The presence of nocturnal erections is consistent with psychogenic E.D., while the absence of nocturnal erections is consistent with organic E.D. However, there are exceptions to this. Men with deep depression do not have nocturnal erections. Additionally, men with sleep disorders, such as sleep apnea, do not experience nocturnal erections. Patients with organic E.D. secondary to a low testosterone level often have reduced but clinically normal nocturnal erections. Thus, this is not a perfect test.

The ideal method to evaluate nocturnal erections is to go to a sleep laboratory. Unfortunately, sleep laboratories are very expensive; they typically cost thousands of dollars each night. In a sleep laboratory, both nocturnal erections and sleep stages are monitored. Thus, in a man who does not have any nocturnal erections, one can document the presence of REM sleep. In the absence of a sleep assessment, it is impossible to state whether the lack of an erection was due to an erection problem or simply because the man did not experience REM sleep that night. At a sleep laboratory, a technician at the site monitors the patient throughout the night (thus, the expense). Once an erection occurs, the technician measures the buckling pressure of the erection, the best measure of penile rigidity. Specifically, a device is used to measure the amount of pressure it takes to buckle, or bend, the penis. This is actually the most clinically relevant measure of an erection. Moreover, the erection can be photographed to provide objective proof, and the patient may be awakened to allow him to assess the quality of his nocturnal erections. Although not perfect, formal sleep laboratory testing provides the best information today as to whether or not a patient has psychogenic or organic E.D.

Nocturnal assessment is necessary to document organic E.D. prior to performing any surgical therapy in a patient in whom a physical problem is not otherwise obvious. In addition, nocturnal testing may be used to convince a man that his E.D. is not physical. Finally, medicolegal issues may require full documentation of the cause of the E.D.

If your health care professional determines that you have E.D., he or she will wish to discuss therapeutic options with you. To learn more about available treatments, including the discovery of Viagra, please see Chapters 6 and 7.

Table 10b

INTERNATIONAL INDEX OF ERECTILE FUNCTION (IIEF)

A MULTIDIMENSIONAL SCALE FOR ASSESSMENT OF ERECTILE DYSFUNCTION

These questions ask about the effects your erection problems have had on your sex life **over the past four weeks**. Please answer the following questions as honestly and clearly as possible. In answering these questions, the following definitions apply:

- **sexual activity** includes intercourse, caressing, foreplay, and masturbation
- **sexual intercourse** is defined as vaginal penetration of the partner (you entered your partner)
- **sexual stimulation** includes situations such as foreplay with a partner, looking at erotic pictures, etc.
- **ejaculate:** the ejection of semen from the penis (or the feeling of this)

1. **Over the past 4 weeks**, how often were you able to get an erection during sexual activity? *Please check one box only.*
    - ❏ No sexual activity
    - ❏ Almost never/never
    - ❏ A few times (much less than half the time)
    - ❏ Sometimes (about half the time)
    - ❏ Most times (much more than half the time)
    - ❏ Almost always/always

2. **Over the past 4 weeks**, when you had erections with sexual stimulation, how often were your erections hard enough for penetration? *Please check one box only.*
    - ❏ No sexual activity
    - ❏ Almost never/never
    - ❏ A few times (much less than half the time)
    - ❏ Sometimes (about half the time)
    - ❏ Most times (much more than half the time)
    - ❏ Almost always/always

The next three questions ask about the erections you may have had during sexual intercourse.

3. Over the past 4 weeks, when you attempted sexual intercourse, how often were you able to penetrate (enter) your partner? *Please check one box only.*
- ❑ No intercourse
- ❑ Almost never/never
- ❑ A few times (much less than half the time)
- ❑ Sometimes (about half the time)
- ❑ Most times (much more than half the time)
- ❑ Almost always/always

4. Over the past 4 weeks, during sexual intercourse, **how often** were you able to maintain your erection after you had penetrated (entered) your partner? *Please check one box only.*
- ❑ Did not attempt intercourse
- ❑ Almost never/never
- ❑ A few times (much less than half the time)
- ❑ Sometimes (about half the time)
- ❑ Most times (much more than half the time)
- ❑ Almost always/always

5. Over the past 4 weeks, during sexual intercourse, **how difficult** was it to maintain your erection to completion of intercourse? *Please check one box only.*
- ❑ Did not attempt intercourse
- ❑ Extremely difficult
- ❑ Very difficult
- ❑ Difficult
- ❑ Slightly difficult
- ❑ Not difficult

6. Over the past 4 weeks, how many times have you attempted sexual intercourse? *Please check one box only.*
- ❑ No attempts
- ❑ One to two attempts
- ❑ Three to four attempts
- ❑ Five to six attempts
- ❑ Seven to ten attempts
- ❑ Eleven or more attempts

7. **Over the past 4 weeks**, when you attempted sexual intercourse, how often was it satisfactory for **you**? *Please check one box only.*
   - ❑ No intercourse
   - ❑ Almost never/never
   - ❑ A few times (much less than half the time)
   - ❑ Sometimes (about half the time)
   - ❑ Most times (much more than half the time)
   - ❑ Almost always/always

8. **Over the past 4 weeks**, how much have you enjoyed sexual intercourse? *Please check one box only.*
   - ❑ No intercourse
   - ❑ No enjoyment
   - ❑ Not very enjoyable
   - ❑ Fairly enjoyable
   - ❑ Highly enjoyable
   - ❑ Very highly enjoyable

9. **Over the past 4 weeks**, when you had sexual stimulation or intercourse, how often did you ejaculate? *Please check one box only.*
   - ❑ No sexual stimulation/intercourse
   - ❑ Almost never/never
   - ❑ A few times (much less than half the time)
   - ❑ Sometimes (about half the time)
   - ❑ Most times (much more than half the time)
   - ❑ Almost always/always

10. **Over the past 4 weeks**, when you had sexual stimulation or intercourse, how often did you have the feeling of orgasm (with or without ejaculation)? *Please check one box only.*
   - ❑ No sexual stimulation/intercourse
   - ❑ Almost never/never
   - ❑ A few times (much less than half the time)
   - ❑ Sometimes (about half the time)
   - ❑ Most times (much more than half the time)
   - ❑ Almost always/always

The next two questions ask about sexual desire. Let's define sexual desire as a feeling that may include wanting to have a sexual experience (for example, masturbation or intercourse), thinking about having sex, or feeling frustrated due to lack of sex.

11. **Over the past 4 weeks**, how often have you felt **sexual desire?** *Please check one box only.*
   ❑ Almost never/never
   ❑ A few times (much less than half the time)
   ❑ Sometimes (about half the time)
   ❑ Most times (much more than half the time)
   ❑ Almost always/always

12. **Over the past 4 weeks**, how would you rate your level of **sexual desire?** *Please check one box only.*
   ❑ Very low or none at all
   ❑ Low
   ❑ Moderate
   ❑ High
   ❑ Very high

13. **Over the past 4 weeks**, how satisfied have you been with your overall **sex life?** *Please check one box only.*
   ❑ Very dissatisfied
   ❑ Moderately dissatisfied
   ❑ About equally satisfied and dissatisfied
   ❑ Moderately satisfied
   ❑ Very satisfied

14. **Over the past 4 weeks**, how satisfied have you been with your **sexual relationship** with your partner? *Please check one box only.*
   ❑ Very dissatisfied
   ❑ Moderately dissatisfied
   ❑ About equally satisfied and dissatisfied
   ❑ Moderately satisfied
   ❑ Very satisfied

15. Over the past 4 weeks, how do you rate your **confidence** that you can get and keep your erection? *Please check one box only*.

❑ Very low
❑ Low
❑ Moderate
❑ High
❑ Very high

Copyright © 1998, Pfizer Inc. Used with permission.

INTERNATIONAL INDEX OF ERECTILE FUNCTION (IIEF)

SCORING ALGORITHM

Subjects should be instructed to complete the IIEF questionnaire by circling *one* response from the response options provided for each of the 15 questions. The response options for each question are scored from 1 to 5, with a score of 0 used to indicate no sexual activity, no intercourse, or no attempts for Questions 1-10 only, as described below.

IIEF Questions	Scoring
Questions 1, 2, 3, 4, 7, 9, and 10	0 = No sexual activity/stimulation/ intercourse 1 = Almost never/never 2 = A few times (much less than half the time) 3 = Sometimes (about half the time) 4 = Most times (much more than half the time) 5 = Almost always/always
Question 5	0 = Did not attempt intercourse 1 = Extremely difficult 2 = Very difficult 3 = Difficult 4 = Slightly difficult 5 = Not difficult
Question 6	0 = No attempts 1 = One to two attempts 2 = Three to four attempts 3 = Five to six attempts 4 = Seven to ten attempts 5 = Eleven or more attempts
Question 8	0 = No intercourse 1 = No enjoyment 2 = Not very enjoyable 3 = Fairly enjoyable 4 = Highly enjoyable 5 = Very highly enjoyable

INTERNATIONAL INDEX OF ERECTILE FUNCTION (IIEF)

IIEF Questions	*Scoring*
Question 11	1 = Almost never/never 2 = A few times (much less than half the time) 3 = Sometimes (about half the time) 4 = Most times (much more than half the time) 5 = Almost always/always
Question 12 and 15	1 = Very low/none at all 2 = Low 3 = Moderate 4 = High 5 = Very High
Question 13 and 14	1 = Very dissatisfied 2 = Moderately dissatisfied 3 = About equally satisfied and dissatisfied 4 = Moderately satisfied 5 = Very satisfied

NOTE: The scores for the 15 questions should be added to determine the overall score.

6

A Decade of Discovery in Pfizer Inc.

The Birth of Viagra

In light of the media attention that Viagra has attracted, one might easily wonder how—and why—did Pfizer Inc discover, or develop, this drug? To begin, it's important to understand and appreciate how the scientific discovery process works. Then, we'll take a look at how drugs in general are discovered, or developed. From there, we'll go on to the specifics of Viagra.

One of the most interesting paperback books we have come across is *Science and Human Values,* written by J. Bronowski and published by Simon & Schuster/Messner, 1956. The three essays in the book were first given as lectures in 1953 by Professor Bronowski at the Massachusetts Institute of Technology, in Cambridge, Massachusetts. His essays exquisitely describe how the scientific community works and what the discovery process is all about. In one passage, for example, Bronowski says that one could trace the start of the Scientific Revolution to 1543, the year that Copernicus's book was published in which he described a thesis he had prepared nearly twelve years earlier—that the earth moved around the sun. From there, a little more than half a century later (somewhere between 1609 and 1619), Bronowski points out that Kepler published the three laws that describe the paths of the planets. Nearly fifty years later, notes Bronowski, Sir Isaac Newton took the idea even further. Bronowski tells the whole story vividly in his essay. To begin, he asks us to recall learning in school about Newton and his "discovery" of gravity. Do you remember that simple tale? Typically, a caricature comes to mind: there's Newton, sitting idly under a tree; an apple falls from it—and presto! Newton comes up with the concept of gravity. Well, that's not quite all there was to it, as Bronowski points out. In fact, prior to this, Newton was studying at the University of Cambridge in England, one of the world's most prestigious universities. Unfortunately, while Newton was there in 1665, the plague broke out in southern England, and the university shut down for more than a year. This frustrated Newton terribly, Bronowski recorded, as Newton wrote: "I was in the prime of my age for invention," and instead, he wound up in his mother's home, waiting for the plague to pass. True enough, one day, while sitting in her garden, Newton watched an apple fall from the tree. But, notes Bronowski, here's where our grade school books don't quite tell us the whole story. What Newton realized, in watching the apple fall to the ground, was *not* simply that the apple is drawn to the earth by gravity; in fact, the concept of gravity was much older than Newton, having been previously established by Copernicus. Rather, Bronowski shows us, what Newton realized was that the same force of gravity that reaches to the top of the tree might reach out well beyond the earth. Newton's *new* thought was this: gravity might reach the moon, and it might well be gravity that holds the moon in orbit. Newton was excited by his hypothesis. Then and there, he worked on the calculations. He took the known force of gravity at tree height, and compared it with what force from the earth would hold the moon. Newton was satisfied that the gravitational forces agreed, and said, "I found the answer pretty nearly."

This vignette, which Bronowski described so thoroughly in his essay, tells the story of modern science: "It grows from comparison," Bronowski observed. In other words, as Bronowski noted, the apple falling from a tree in a summer garden and the gold moon in the ink-black sky overhead are about as unlike in their movements as any two objects can be. But Isaac Newton traced in these two objects—the apple and the moon— "two expressions of a single concept, gravitation," and that, Bronowski wrote, is how science progresses: "Unity comes to what had long seemed unlike."*

Interestingly enough, in 1796, Edward Jenner—like Newton—linked the unlike with the like and triggered a new voyage of discovery in medical

*Adapted with the permission of Simon & Schuster from *Science and Human Values* by J. Bronowski, ©1956, 1965 by J. Bronowski; copyright renewed 1984, 1993 by Rita Bronowski.

management of diseases. Jenner's approach was to use a disease—the cowpox virus—to inoculate people against disease—the smallpox virus. At the time, his approach, or discovery, which we consider common-place today, changed the course of medical therapy forever.

Another book, first published in 1977, is also very helpful in under-standing medical pathways to progress. The book, *Retrospectroscope*, written by Julius H. Comroe, Jr., a well known medical researcher and educator who spent approximately sixteen years as director of the Uni-versity of California's rather large Cardiovascular Research Institute in San Francisco, explores insights into medical discoveries. In the preface to his book, Comroe says that he wrote the book to "determine how recent life-saving advances in some branches of medicine and surgery had actually come about." To summarize, Comroe shows us what Bronowski has already told us: scientists depend on the work of other scientists, who depend on the work of still others. In one analysis of published research papers, for example, Comroe et al showed that, over-all, 41 percent of medical investigators reported work that, at the time it was done, had no relationship *whatsoever* to the disease that it later helped to prevent, diagnose, alleviate, or treat. To appreciate this, Comroe gives us some examples. For one, researcher Sidney Ringer was at work study-ing a basic physiologic problem in frogs when he realized that, in proper proportions, potassium and calcium ions were critical to maintaining normal heart rhythm and normal heart muscle contractions (the con-tractions help "pump" the blood continuously through the heart). At the time of his work, Comroe points out, Ringer had *no* idea that his work would help others subsequently understand the relationship be-tween electrolyte disturbances and cardiac abnormalities in humans (*e.g.*, if you lose too much potassium from your body, a cardiac arrhythmia, or irregular heartbeat, can develop). His work also proved to be clinically important in elective cardiac arrest during open heart surgery, and in the development and use of a cardiac defibrillator.

Comroe cites another example of how one scientific "discovery" leads to another—planned or not; it's the story of the discovery of x-rays. Wilhelm Conrad Roentgen, professor of physics at the University of Wurzberg——who, in fact, coined the term "x-ray"—was a physicist exploring a basic problem: how to deal with the electrical nature of mat-ter. As Comroe writes, Roentgen was at work in his laboratory in 1894 and 1895; he had not set out to determine how to "look inside" people. Still, in the course of his studies, he found that rays from a Crookes tube (a type of glass tube) could, indeed, pass through a human hand and darken photographic plates. With this realization, the simple x-ray, as we've come to know it, was born. In 1896, shortly after Roentgen presented his paper on his work, there was relatively quick and widespread application of this newly discovered technology. Comroe notes, for example, that anatomists could now view the human skeleton, without the patient ever even having to undress! Doctors could now see the broken bones they had to set, and, just two years after Roentgen's discovery, Comroe tells us that W.S. Hedley published a survey of how the new technology was being applied to nonmedical problems. He reported that gemologists, for instance, were using the x-ray technique to help them distinguish real gems from fake ones, whereas others had applied x-ray technology to view the contents of parcel post packages, something that even Comroe himself thought was unique to our present-day culture!

To appreciate the impact of the discovery of x-ray technology even more, Comroe quoted the first presidential address given before the Roentgen Society in November 1897, by Sylvanus Thompson. In his remarks, Thompson said:

> In the history of Science, nothing is more true than the discoverer—even the greatest of discoverers—is but the descendant of his scientific forefathers, is always and essentially the product of the age in which he was born. Roentgen himself has frankly avowed the ancestry of his discoveries. He himself has stated that, being aware of the existence of unsolved problems respecting the emission of cathode rays in and by an electrically stimulated vacuum tube, he had for a long time followed with the greatest interest the researchers of Hertz and of Lenard, and had determined, as soon as he should find the necessary leisure, to make some researches of his own. Behind Roentgen, stand Lenard and Hertz; behind Hertz stand Crookes, and Varley, and Hittorf, and Sprengel and Geissler; and so back to Hauksbee, and Boyle, and Otto Guericke, into the beginnings of modern science as it emerged from the vain imaginings and occult mysteries of Mediaeval night.

In that address, Thompson also observed:

> Roentgen's discovery cannot in any sense be called accidental; it was the result of deliberate and directed thought. He was looking for something— *he knew not precisely what.* And he found it. Fortunate the discovery may well be deemed, but not fortuitous.

Comroe then poses the question: Could someone else have discovered the x-ray? Comroe pointed out that Crookes could have come up with it earlier; he had developed some photographic plates after experimenting with his tube, and he had also seen marks on his pictures that corresponded to his fingers. But, noted Comroe, Crookes had thought the plates were defective and fired off a nasty letter to the manufacturer—and returned them!

Comroe's text saves one of the most interesting scientific considerations for last. X-ray therapy, he notes, was first reported to *cure* cancer in 1899, three years *before* the first report of x-rays *causing* cancer was published. And thus, he leaves us to think about this: "If the cancer-*caused* had preceded the cancer-*cured*, would the story of x-rays have stopped abruptly with the cancer-caused?"*

As much as it may surprise you, then, the discovery of Viagra is also just another link in the long, winding chain of the scientific, or medical discovery, process. Was Pfizer working on a cure for E.D. when their researchers developed the compound sildenafil citrate? No more so than Professor Roentgen set out to create a whole new medical technology by pursuing his research interest: the electrical nature of matter.

The Discovery of Viagra

The story of Viagra's discovery begins in one of the three main research facilities of Pfizer Inc in Sandwich, in the United Kingdom (the other two facilities are located in Groton, Connecticut, and Nagaya, Japan). There, a group of well-trained physicians and scientists work in laboratories creating chemical compounds and consider their viability to treat a disease, to detect a medical disorder, and so forth. At present, Pfizer's research and development program has over 170 research projects underway.

For more than fifteen years Pfizer Inc. has been one of the leading pharmaceutical manufacturers in cardiovascular drugs (see "Highlights in the History of Pfizer Inc., in this chapter). The company currently manufactures several major cardiovascular medicines that are routinely used today: Procardia XL® (nifedipine), Norvasc® (amlodipine), and Cardura® (doxazosin). All of these drugs are used to treat specific types

---

*Excerpted from *Retrospectroscope: Insight Into medical Discovery*, by Julius H. Comroe, Jr., published in 1977 by Von Gehr Press. Permission granted by the sole distributor, Perinatalogy Press, Ithaca, NY 14851.

of heart disease, such as angina and hypertension. Norvasc, for instance, is one of the most commonly prescribed antihypertensives worldwide today. Because of their strong expertise in cardiovascular medicine, it was natural for Pfizer researchers to continue to look for newer, even better cardiovascular drugs. To that end, in or about 1986, the Pfizer laboratory scientists working in Sandwich developed a new chemical compound, sildenafil citrate, and considered it a candidate for the treatment of angina. In order to determine whether or not this agent could be used effectively to treat angina, however, the company, like all drug companies, tested the drug very rigorously; typically, in three phases (see "How a Drug Is Tested Before You Buy It," in this chapter).

After seven studies, giving sildenafil several times a day to test subjects, the Pfizer researchers soon recognized that its effect on heart disease was not as significant as they had hoped. But the researchers observed another effect of sildenafil: many patients experienced restored erectile function. The researchers wondered: Is sexual health linked to the vasculature in a manner that can simply be treated with a pill?—and, if so, how? At first, the researchers thought the erections were a fluke; at this critical juncture, Pfizer could have missed the boat. Today, in light of the avalanche of publicity that surrounded Viagra's introduction to the market, it's probably very difficult for you to imagine that a drug company could ignore exploring this effect of the drug. But remember Crookes? He was so busy being angry at the manufacturers of his "defective" photographic plates that he *did* miss out on "discovering" the x-ray! Also, keep in mind that Pfizer was pursuing development of another cardiovascular drug. Fortunately, the team of Pfizer researchers, headed by Ian Osterloh, M.D., and the company's management decided to allocate staff and resources to continue the investigation of sildenafil's potential in the treatment of E.D.

During this time, another group of academic researchers published a paper which revealed that, during sexual stimulation, nonadrenergic, noncholinergic nerves in the penis release nitric oxide which, in turn, causes an increase in the levels of cGMP in the penis. As was discussed in Chapter 3, elevated cGMP levels are largely responsible for the smooth muscle relaxation that is necessary for an erection (see Figure 13). The Pfizer researchers' approach to investigating the effects of sildenafil echoes that of Newton's approach: the researchers took two apparently unrelated disorders—heart disease and E.D.—and viewed them through a single enzyme, PDE_5. Their scientific quest led to the discovery of the first approved oral medication proven effective for E.D.

Figure 13. How VIAGRA works to help you achieve and maintain an erection

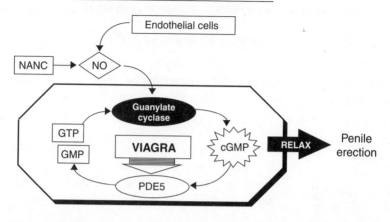

NO is released from neurons and endothelial cells (lining the arteries), increasing the amount of smooth muscle cGMP. Increased levels of cGMP are involved in smooth muscle relaxation; this, in turn, leads to penile erection. Next, cGMP is converted back to GMP by PDE_5. Viagra is a highly selective inhibitor of PDE_5 and prevents the breakdown of cGMP; thus, premature loss of erection does not occur.

NO = nitric oxide	GMP = guanosine monophase
NANC = nonadrenergic-noncholinergic neurons	cGMP = cyclic guanosine monophase
GTP = guanosine triphosphate	PDE5 = phosphodiesterase type 5

Adapted with permission from Ignarro, L.J., et al. *J Pharmacol Exp Ther.* 1981; 281: 739–749

Shortly thereafter, the clinical trials began; now more than 3,000 men worldwide, ages nineteen to eighty-seven, have taken Viagra; up to 82 percent of them have reported erections satisfactory for sexual intercourse, compared with only 20 percent on placebo. We mentioned earlier how it is currently estimated that E.D. affects more than 100 million men and their partners worldwide, but less than 10 percent of these men seek treatment—either due to embarrassment or to the lack of noninvasive and effective treatment options. Today, for the first time in the history of modern medicine, patients suffering with E.D. have an effective oral medication for the treatment of E.D. Results of the studies showed that Viagra is highly effective, reliable, fast-acting, well-tolerated, and natural; it works only in response to sexual stimulation. The studies also showed that Viagra is effective in a wide range of patients: diabetics, patients treated for hypertension, patients with spinal cord injury, prostatectomies, depression, and/or E.D. due to psychogenic origin. Viagra is also effective in all age groups, including elderly patients and patients with mild-to-severe E.D.

Table 11

A MILESTONE IN MEDICINE: THE DEVELOPMENT OF VIAGRA

1981–1983	Increasing medical evidence links E.D. to physical causes.
1985	Development of injection treatments sheds new light on E.D.
1990	Pfizer tests sildenafil.
1992	Results of using sildenafil in angina are disappointing, but some men report unexpected incidence of erections. Pfizer researchers study the link between sildenafil and enhanced blood flow to the penis.
	During this time, academic researchers describe the role of nitric oxide in penile blood flow.
1993	Pfizer researchers in Sandwich, United Kingdom, initiate the first clinical studies of Viagra for E.D.
1994–1995	Results of initial studies look promising; Pfizer informs opinion-leading E.D. researchers of initial trial results.
1995	The International Index of Erectile Function (IIEF), a scientifically validated patient questionnaire to assess E.D., is developed; Pfizer provides support for development and validation of the tool. Phase II Viagra studies demonstrate impressive efficacy; large-scale Viagra research trials include patients with E.D. associated with numerous medical conditions, including diabetes and high blood pressure.
1996	Viagra data is published in *British Medical Journal* and *Journal of Impotence Research*.
1998	The U.S. Food and Drug Administration grants market clearance for Viagra, a breakthrough oral treatment for E.D. on March 27, 1998.

Adopted from the press kit, VIAGRA™ (sildenafil citrate), ©1998 Pfizer Inc., with permission.

In late March 1998, shortly before the U.S. Food and Drug Administration approved Viagra for use, the television program "20/20" aired a report on Viagra; in it, a young man with a spinal cord injury, confined to a wheelchair, told of his experience with the drug. Among other things, he pointed out, he would now be able to have a family.

Certainly, we recognize that Viagra is in a class by itself because it is the first effective oral medication approved for the treatment of E.D. (see Table 11). But is Viagra the *only* drug that started out being tested for

---

HIGHLIGHTS IN THE HISTORY OF PFIZER INC, THE MAKERS OF VIAGRA

When Charles Pfizer started a pharmacy in Brooklyn, New York, in 1858, he probably never imagined that his company would turn out as it has! In a little more than a hundred years, the small plant in Brooklyn has mushroomed into the research-based, global health care company that we know today as Pfizer Inc. Overall, the blue-chip, Fortune 500 company has three key business segments: health care, consumer health care, and animal health. Pfizer develops innovative products that help improve the quality of life of people around the world. Currently, Pfizer products are available in 150 countries. The company's revenue for 1997 was approximately $12.5 billion.

Although it may not be widely known, Pfizer's Consumer Health Care Group is a worldwide marketer of leading over-the-counter products, such as Desitin® for diaper rash treatment, Visine® (eye drops), and BenGay® for topical analgesic relief. The Animal Health Care Group is among the largest in the world and is the leading supplier of vaccines for cattle. Pfizer's portfolio of prescription drugs also lists some of the most effective and widely prescribed medications in the U.S. and in many other countries, including the antihypertensive Norvasc® (amlodipine), antibiotics Zithromax® (azithromycin) and Trovan® (trovafloxacin), and the world's largest-selling prescription antifungal: Diflucan®. With Viagra, Pfizer enters the sexual health care arena in a significant way, but Viagra is not Pfizer's first "breakthrough." In fact, a half-century ago, Charles Pfizer & Company achieved one of the most important medical breakthroughs of this century—a revolutionary process for the mass production of penicillin, a true "wonder drug."

Since 1991, Pfizer has jumped from the number thirteen position to number four in global prescription sales. The goal now is for Pfizer to be the number one health care company by 2001. The successful development of Viagra may help them reach that goal.

one disorder and ended up being effective for another indication? Definitely not. Minoxidil, for example, is another drug in which one of its effects, in fact, became the treatment. Initially, minoxidil was used as an antihypertensive drug, but it also had the effect of causing hirsutism (excess hair growth). The drug is still used today to treat high blood pressure, but the manufacturers also pursued another avenue; i.e., minoxidil's effect on hair growth. It was subsequently developed in a topical formulation (2 percent for both men and women and, recently, 5

HOW A DRUG IS TESTED BEFORE YOU USE IT

An investigational new drug application may be submitted for one or more phases of an investigation. The clinical investigation of a previously untested drug is generally divided into three phases. Although, in general, the phases are conducted sequentially, they may overlap. The three phases of an investigation are:

Phase I: Phase I includes the initial introduction of an investigational new drug into humans. Phase I studies are typically monitored and may be conducted in patients or normal volunteer subjects. These studies are designed to determine the metabolism and pharmacologic actions of the drug in humans, the side effects associated with increasing doses, and early evidence on effectiveness (if possible). During Phase I, sufficient information about the drug's pharmacokinetics and pharmacologic effects should be obtained to permit the design of well-controlled, scientifically valid Phase II studies. The total number of subjects and patients included in Phase I studies varies with the drug, but is generally in the range of twenty to eighty.

Phase II: Phase II includes the controlled clinical studies conducted to evaluate the effectiveness of the drug for a particular indication or indications in patients with the disease or condition under study, to determine the common short-term side effects and risks associated with the drug. Phase II studies are typically well controlled, closely monitored, and conducted in a relatively small number of patients, usually involving no more than several hundred subjects.

Phase III: Phase III studies are expanded controlled and uncontrolled trials. They are performed after preliminary evidence suggesting effectiveness of the drug has been obtained, and are intended to gather the additional information about effectiveness and safety that is needed to evaluate the overall benefit-risk relationship of the drug as well as to provide an adequate basis for physician labeling. Phase III studies usually include from several hundred to several thousand subjects.

percent for men only) to regrow hair for baldness. Today, this is minoxidil's most prevalent use.

Sometimes, too, "folk" knowledge and practices lead to drug development. For example, today it is estimated that approximately 25 percent of drugs in use come from various plant sources. What took the scientists and medical researchers to plants in the first place? Again, it's all part of the scientific discovery process! Botanists studying plants for one set of reasons stumble upon findings that they realize may be useful to medical researchers, and vice versa. In fact, due to the interrelationship between the study of plants and drug development, several of the large pharmaceutical companies, including Pfizer Inc, provide very substantial support to some of the major botanical gardens around the world, so that the botanists and other investigators there can pursue numerous avenues of research (see Table 12).

Now, back to Viagra. To find out more about whether or not Viagra is, indeed, a "wonder drug," please go on to Chapter 7.

Table 12

FIFTY DRUGS DISCOVERED FROM PLANT SOURCES

Below is a list of some commonly used drugs that are derived from plant sources. Overall, approximately 45 percent of drugs in use today are derived from plant sources.

DRUG	MEDICAL USE	PLANT SPECIES
Ajmaline	Heart arrhythmia	*Rauvolfia spp.*
Aspirin	Analgesic, inflammation	*Filipendula ulmaria*
Atropine	Ophthalmology	*Atropa belladonna*
Benzoin	Oral disinfectant	*Styrax tonkinensis*
Caffeine	Stimulant	*Camellia sinensis*
Camphor	Rheumatic pain	*Cinnamomum camphora*
Cascara	Purgative	*Rhamnus purshiana*
Cocaine	Ophthalmologic anaesthetic	*Erythroxylum coca*
Codeine	Analgesic, antitussive	*Papaver somniferum*
Colchicine	Gout	*Colchicum autumnale*
Demecolcine	Leukemia, lymphomata	*Colchicum autumnale*
Deserpidine	Hypertension	*Rauvolfia canescens*
Dicoumarol	Thrombosis	*Melilotus officinalis*
Digitoxin	Atrial fibrillation	*Digitalis purpurea*
Digoxin	Atrial fibrillation	*Digitalis purpurea*
Emetine	Amoebic dysentery	*Cephaelis ipecachuanha*
Ephedrine	Bronchodilator	*Ephedra sinica*
Eugenol	Toothache	*Syzygium aromaticum*
Gallotanins	Hemorrhoid suppository	*Hamamelis virginiana*
Hyoscyamine	Anticholinergic	*Hyoscyamus niger*
Ipecac	Emetic	*Cephaelis ipecacuanha*
Ipratropium	Bronchodilator	*Hyoscyamus niger*
Morphine	Analgesic	*Papaver somniferum*

Table 12 (*continued*)

50 DRUGS DISCOVERED FROM PLANT SOURCES

DRUG	MEDICAL USE	PLANT SPECIES
Noscapine	Antitussive	*Papaver somniferum*
Papain	Attenuates mucus	*Carica papaya*
Papaverine	Antispasmodic	*Papaver somniferum*
Physostigmine	Glaucoma	*Physostigma venenosum*
Picrotoxin	Barbiturate antidoe	*Anamirta cocculus*
Pilocarpine	Glaucoma	*Pilocarpus jaborandi*
Podophyllotoxin	Condylomata acuminata	*Podophyllum peltatum*
Proscillaridin	Cardiac malfunction	*Drimia maritima*
Protoveratine	Hypertension	*Veratrum album*
Pseudoephedrine	Rhinitis	*Ephedra sinica*
Psoralen	Vitiligo	*Psoralea corylifolia*
Quinidine	Cardiac arrhythmia	*Cinchona pubescens*
Quinine	Malaria prophylaxis	*Cinchona pubescens*
Rescinnamine	Hypertension	*Rauvolfia serpentina*
Reserpine	Hypertension	*Rauvolfia serpentina*
Sennoside A,B	Laxative	*Cassia angustifolia*
Scopolamine	Motion sickness	*Datura stramonium*
Stigmasterol	Steroidal precursor	*Physostigma venenosum*
Strophanthin	Congestive heart failure	*Strophanthus gratus*
Teniposide	Bladder neoplasms	*Podophyllum peltatum*
THC	Antiemetic	*Cannabis sativa*
Theophylline	Diuretic, asthma	*Camellia sinensis*
Toxiferine	Surgery, relaxant	*Strychnos guianensis*
Tubocurarine	Muscle relaxant	*Chondrodendron tomentosum*
Vinblastine	Hodgkin's disease	*Ctharanthus roseus*
Vincristine	Pediatric leukemia	*Ctharanthus roseus*
Xanthotoxin	Vitiligo	*Ammi majus*

From *Plants, People, and Culture: The Science of Ethnobotany*, by Balick and Cox, ©1996 by Scientific American Library. Used with permission of W.H. Freeman and Company.

7

Viagra
Is It a Wonder Drug?

What's in a name? Just say "Viagra." The very sound of it—Viagra—evokes power and life.

Viagra is the brand name for the medication sildenafil citrate. Viagra is the first oral pill ever approved to treat male E.D. It was approved by the U.S. Food and Drug Administration (FDA) for doctors to prescribe on March 27, 1998. Since then, the drug has received an avalanche of publicity, and over 2.5 million American men have visited their physicians to discuss this new treatment for E.D., and more than 3.6 million prescriptions have been written.

But what was life like for most men who suffered with E.D. prior to the introduction of Viagra? Up until earlier this year, any treatment for E.D. was awkward, embarrassing, and often uncomfortable. In other cases, the only solution was surgery, an option that many men understandably avoided.

What did these older therapies involve? Specifically, treatments for E.D. had been limited to injecting drugs directly into the penis, inserting suppositories into the urethra, using a vacuum device to draw blood into the penis, and surgical procedures, such as implantation of penile prostheses. In this setting, the unique advantage of Viagra is obvious: it is a small pill, taken orally approximately one hour prior to sexual activity, and it is highly effective in many men, resulting in an erection satisfactory for sexual intercourse.

How Does Viagra Work?

In order to comprehend how Viagra works, one must understand the basics of how an erection works, which we discussed in detail in Chapter 3. To review briefly, you will recall that during sexual stimulation a substance called nitric oxide (NO) is released by nerves and cells lining the blood vessels in the spongy erectile tissue of the penis, called the corpus cavernosum. NO activates an enzyme called guanylate cyclase, which causes an increase in the substance cyclic guanosine monophosphate (cGMP); cGMP is a key factor in causing an erection because it relaxes the smooth muscle cells in the erectile tissue of the penis, thereby allowing blood to rush into this spongy tissue. At this point, the penis stiffens, and a man has an erection. Men with E.D. often lack sufficient cGMP. Viagra *enhances* the levels of cGMP in erectile tissue by inhibiting another enzyme that breaks down cGMP, which can result in loss of an erection. This enzyme is called phosphodiesterase type 5, or PDE_5. Viagra works by blocking, or inhibiting, PDE_5 so cGMP remains at a level consistent to maintain an erection (see Figure 14).

Figure 14. How VIAGRA works to help you achieve and maintain an erection

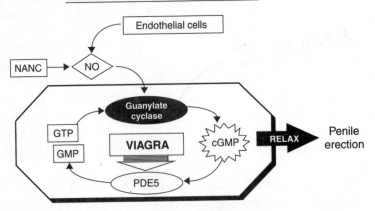

NO is released from neurons and endothelial cells (lining the arteries), increasing the amount of smooth muscle cGMP. Increased levels of cGMP are involved in smooth muscle relaxation; this, in turn, leads to penile erection. Next, cGMP is converted back to GMP by PDE_5. Viagra is a highly selective inhibitor of PDE_5 and prevents the breakdown of cGMP; thus, premature loss of erection does not occur.

NO = nitric oxide
NANC = nonadrenergic-noncholinergic neurons
GTP = guanosine triphosphate

GMP = guanosine monophase
cGMP = cyclic guanosine monophase
PDE5 = phosphodiesterase type 5

Adapted with permission from Ignarro, L.J., et al. *J Pharmacol Exp Ther.* 1981; 281: 739–749

The beauty of Viagra's chemical effect is that it enhances a man's *natural response* to sexual stimulation. In other words, proper use of Viagra makes it easier to obtain an erection, but sexual stimulation *must* occur. At this juncture, we should emphasize a key point about Viagra that's worth repeating: Viagra is not a sexual stimulant itself, and it is *not* an aphrodisiac. Viagra will not increase libido or your desire to engage in sexual activity, so it's not advisable to turn to this medication to help you if a loss of desire is the problem. Also, it's important to keep in mind that in the absence of sexual stimulation taking Viagra will not result in an erection. Actually, this is good news because most men don't want to walk around with an erection outside of the bedroom. Some of the other therapies for E.D. can cause an erection without sexual stimulation, and that can leave a man in the very uncomfortable position of experiencing an erection when he doesn't want one. To understand more about how Viagra works, it is important to know how a medication works within your body. Keep in mind, too, that factors such as age, sex, weight, and the presence of concomitant diseases can also affect not only how a drug works, but how it interacts with other drugs.

Before we turn our attention specifically to Viagra, let's look at the factors that *all* drugs have in common: it's called the pharmacodynamic/pharmacokinetic profile. To make this easy to understand, we will simply call it the drug profile.

What Is a Drug Profile?

For the purposes of this book, we only need to look at a few key factors in the drug profile (see Figure 15). These factors are:

- absorption
- clearance
- excretion
- metabolism

Understanding these features of a drug is useful because it will help you appreciate why Viagra works. Also, you'll see why your physician has to ask you about any other medications you are taking, including over-the-counter medications, in order to ensure that no adverse drug-drug interactions will occur.

Figure 15. <u>Key factors in a drug profile</u>

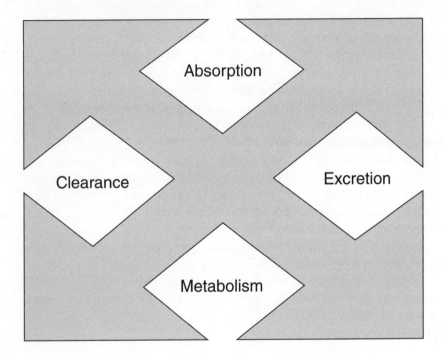

Absorption: When you take a drug orally, it is absorbed into your body through the intestinal tract. The term *absorption* refers to how a substance or drug is absorbed into the bloodstream and tissues throughout the body after it is ingested (taken). Once the drug is absorbed into the bloodstream from the gastrointestinal tract, its concentration in the bloodstream peaks; this is the point at which you generally begin to experience the effects of the drug.

Clearance: Your body naturally clears what you ingest—foods, beverages, and medications. The term *clearance* specifically refers to how a substance or drug is removed from the tissues and bloodstream. Many drugs are broken down by enzymes in the liver and other tissues. Usually the breakdown products are then excreted through one or more routes, such as urine, feces, or both.

Excretion: This function refers to the elimination or discharge of the drug or its breakdown products. Drugs and their breakdown products can be excreted through bile, a fluid that is secreted by the liver into the intestine and eliminated through the stool, or the drug may be excreted through the kidney in urine.

Metabolism: This term describes the myriad chemical processes by which the body transforms foodstuffs and substances such as drugs into available substances your body can use—for energy, healing, and so forth.

Viagra is metabolized, or broken down in the body, by specific enzymes, most of which are in the liver. Certain drugs, such as a medication commonly used to treat ulcers, Tagamet® (cimetidine), and the frequently prescribed antibiotic erythromycin, block or inhibit these enzymes, thereby decreasing the breakdown of Viagra; thus, higher levels of Viagra remain in your body. Other drugs, too, such as antifungals, can also reduce the body's ability to clear Viagra. Because of this, if you take these medications, your physician may reduce the dose of Viagra prescribed to you so you can comfortably remain on the other medications.

On the other hand, at least one drug—an antibiotic called rifampin, which is given to treat tuberculosis—may have the opposite effect; that is, its use stimulates the enzymes that break down Viagra, thereby reducing the blood levels of Viagra in your system. In this setting, your doctor may recommend increasing your dose of Viagra if you also need to take this drug.

There are several other commonly used drugs which, although they affect absorption and drug levels of other drugs, do *not* affect Viagra. For example, magnesium or aluminum-based antacids such as Mylanta®, Phillips Milk of Magnesia® and some forms of Maalox®, do not affect the absorption of Viagra. Similarly, tolbutamide (an oral blood glucose lowering drug used to manage diabetes) and warfarin (a blood thinner), also have no effect on Viagra levels.

In addition, many very common medications used to treat garden-variety hypertension, such as thiazide diuretics (a type of "water pill"), angiotensin converting enzyme (ACE) inhibitors, and calcium channel blockers—such as Norvasc—do *not* interact with Viagra. Lastly, frequently prescribed antidepressants, called selective serotonin reuptake inhibitors (SSRIs), such as Prozac® and Zoloft®, and the older tricyclic antidepressants, do not interact with Viagra. Thus, patients can take any of these medications comfortably while also using Viagra.

Finally—and more good news—Viagra does not interact with aspirin, alcohol, or other common over-the-counter medications. Still, we do not recommend using alcohol with *any* drug, including over-the-counter products. It is possible that, as of the time of this writing, there are other drugs that interact with Viagra, but their interactions are unknown. There is some concern that Viagra could interact with protease inhibitors (anti-AIDS drugs) because they are both broken down by the same liver enzyme. As such, patients on protease inhibitors may need to start on a lower dose of Viagra. Tests are currently underway to investigate this issue as well as other potential drug-drug interactions.

How Effective Is Viagra?

To find out whether or not Viagra could restore satisfactory erections in men with E.D., medical investigators organized a series of clinical studies. Their goal was to evaluate men with E.D. due to both organic or psychogenic causes, to see if use of Viagra would improve each man's ability to develop an erection, provided sexual stimulation also occurred. The researchers used a technique called penile plethysmography, which measures increases in rigidity and engorgement, or swelling of the penis. These effects were measured after one hour of an oral dose of Viagra. In one group of men, the increase in erectile response was still present four hours after taking a dose of Viagra, but the response at four hours was not as great as it was at two hours.

Worldwide: The First 3,000 Men on Viagra

In the twenty-one clinical studies with Viagra, men with E.D. were given a tablet of Viagra or a placebo; then, their ability to achieve and maintain an erection sufficient for sexual activity was determined. Each patient was also given a questionnaire and asked two key questions regarding his ability to achieve and maintain an erection sufficient for sexual intercourse. In these double-blind, placebo-controlled studies, Viagra was given to men in doses of 25 mg, 50 mg, and 100 mg for up to six months. A double-blind, placebo-controlled study means the following: first, neither the patient *nor* the physicians administering the pills knew whether or not each patient was being given an actual tablet of Viagra, or a placebo ("dummy" pill). This is important since this type of study must control for a placebo effect, which is a small, beneficial effect that may occur, even though the patient has only taken the placebo. At the end of the study, the codes are broken and both doctors and patients learn who received Viagra and who took the placebo pills. Overall, the medicine was given to more than 3,000 male patients worldwide, ranging in ages from nineteen to eighty-seven years. Of these, more than 500 were treated for longer than one year. All of the men in the studies suffered from E.D. due to various causes—psychologic as well as organic diseases—and each man had reported a history of E.D. for an average of five years.

Astounding Study Results

The results of these studies were astounding, indicating that medical researchers were on the verge of an exciting breakthrough in the treatment of E.D. Specifically, the investigators discovered that Viagra, even at the lowest dose of one 25 mg pill, significantly improved erectile function in nearly two-thirds of the men in the study. When the dose of Viagra was increased to one 50 mg pill, rather than 25 mg, 74 percent of men reported improvement in their erections; that number jumped to 82 percent of men reporting their erections improved when the dose of Viagra was increased to 100 mg (see Figure 16). On the other hand, only 24 percent of patients taking a placebo reported an erection. The results of these studies were crystal clear: appropriate use of Viagra in men with a history of E.D. was highly effective, and statistically significant when compared with the placebo.

Patient Diaries: But there was even more to learn from these studies! In some of the trials, for example, the patients also kept diaries. When the medical researchers analyzed approximately 1,600 of these patient diaries, they discovered that Viagra had no effect at all on how often the patients attempted to have intercourse (the average was two times per week), but there was an improvement in sexual function, with average success rates of 1.3 successful attempts at sex per week on the 50–100 mg dose versus a success rate of only 0.4 times per week on the placebo. The mean success rate for sexual intercourse was 66 percent on Viagra, compared with only about 20 percent on placebo.

In another study, the female partners of the men corroborated improved erections on Viagra. With this number of rigorous clinical studies on Viagra completed, the researchers then turned their attention to

Figure 16. VIAGRA Efficacy: (improvement in erections)

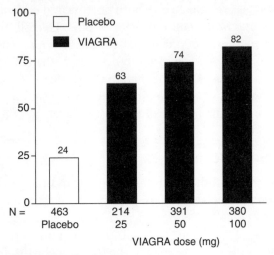

Overall treatment p<0.0001 VIAGRA vs placebo.

From: Viagra® (sildenafil citrate) tablets — Product Monograph © Pfizer Inc. July, 1998. Reprinted with permission. Data on file, Pfizer Inc.

evaluating the impact of side effects from Viagra on patients. The researchers set up open-label studies, lasting for up to one year—an open-label study simply means that the patient knows what medication he or she is taking; in this case, Viagra. In these studies, few men withdrew from treatment with Viagra for any reason, including lack of efficacy. In fact, at the end of the analysis, nearly 90 percent of the men reported improvements in their erections, as a direct result of taking Viagra.

Thus far, we have only seen a few full-length papers published in medical journals regarding the effectiveness of Viagra, although several more are in press. One of the first such papers was published in the prestigious *British Journal of Urology* in 1996. In that study, investigators used objective measures of erectile function by measuring penile plethysmography in men with E.D. After visual sexual stimulation, the mean duration of erections was approximately one minute with placebo, seven to eight minutes with 25 mg of Viagra, and eight to eleven minutes with 50 mg of Viagra. These men also kept diaries of E.D. after taking a placebo, compared with 25 mg of Viagra once daily over seven days. The number of successful erections with satisfactory sexual activity was about five times greater with Viagra, as compared with the placebo (see Figure 17 on the next page).

Figure 17. <u>The patients' diaries reflected the average number of grade 3 and 4 erections, with time after single doses of either VIAGRA or placebo.</u>

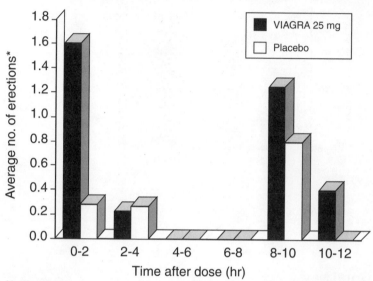

N=12 patients.
*As recorded in patients' diaries; the peaks at 8-10 hours after dosing represent early morning erections.

<u>Grading of penile erectile response</u>

1. Increase in size of penis but no hardness

2. Increase in size and slight increase in hardness (rigidity), but insufficient for sexual intercourse

3. Increase in hardness (rigidity) sufficient for sexual intercourse, but not fully rigid

4. Fully rigid erection

Reproduced with permission from Boolell M, Gepi-Attee S, Gingell JC, Allen MJ. Sildenafil, a novel effective oral therapy for male erectile dysfunction. Br J Urol. 1996;78:257-261.

**Figure 18. The number of successful attempts at sexual intercourse
per month was higher among men receiving VIAGRA**

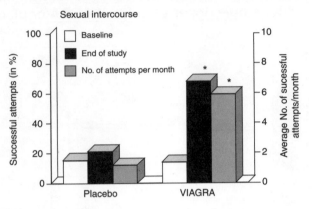

*p<0.001 vs placebo.

Reprinted with permission from Goldstein I, Lue TF, Padma-nathan H, Rosen RC, Steers WD, Wicker PA, for the
sildenafil study group. Oral Sildenafil in the Treatment of Erectile Dysfunction. *N Engl J Med.* 1998; 338: 1397–1402.

More Good News:
A Report in The New England Journal of Medicine

To shed even more light on the effectiveness of Viagra, a rigorous study
was carried out and the results published in The *New England Journal of
Medicine,* one of the most prestigious medical peer-review journals worldwide. Actually, the article, "Oral Sildenafil (Viagra) in the Treatment of
E rectile Dysfunction," discusses two studies in one. The first double-
blind study was a 24-week, dose-response study of 532 men with E.D.
The average age of the men was fifty-seven to fifty-eight years old; the
average history of their E.D. was 3.2 years. The men had E.D. of organic,
psychogenic, or combined origin. The effect of Viagra was determined
for each man by having him fill out a standard questionnaire—the International Index of Erectile Function (IIEF), which was discussed in detail in Chapter 5. Question three of this questionnaire asks: "When you
attempted sexual intercourse, how often were you able to penetrate (enter) your partner?" Question four asks: "During sexual intercourse, how
often were you able to maintain your erection after you had penetrated
(entered) your partner?" In the study, 532 men were randomly assigned

to take a fixed dose of placebo, or 25, 50, or 100 mg of Viagra about one hour before planned sexual activity over a 24-week time period. The men were also instructed to fill out the questionnaires at the beginning of the study, and at twelve and twenty-four weeks. In this study, Viagra clearly improved erections; increasing the doses up to 100 mg was associated with the best responses. In fact, the highest dose (100 mg) resulted in a mean score for the question about achieving erections that was 100 percent greater than at baseline, or before receiving the medicine. In addition, the highest dose, at 100 mg, also resulted in a mean score for the question about maintaining erection of 3.9 versus 1.7 at baseline. At twenty-four weeks, 56 percent, 77 percent, and 84 percent of men taking the 25-, 50-, and 100-mg dose (respectively) reported improved erections, versus only 25 percent of men on placebo.

The authors of the paper, all professors from major university medical centers, and one physician from Pfizer's research center in Groton, Connecticut, reported the results of a second study. That trial was a 12-week, flexible dose-escalation protocol. Overall, 329 men participated; the average age of the men was fifty-nine to sixty years; the average history of E.D. was 4.7 to 5.0 years. First, the men were randomly assigned to take a placebo or Viagra, at 50 mg, one hour before sexual activity. During the study, the men were seen at follow-up visits, and it was their responsibility to talk to their physician about doubling the dose, or alternatively, reducing the dose to 25 mg, depending upon their experiences over the weeks with Viagra at 50 mg. The men filled out the International Index of Erectile Function form at the beginning of the study, and again at twelve weeks, and were asked about the overall, or global, effectiveness of the drug. Men who completed this portion of the study and who did not have any serious side effects were eligible to receive Viagra in an "open-label" study fashion; that is, going forward, they would know that they were taking Viagra, not a placebo. These men then continued on Viagra for thirty-two additional weeks.

In this study, the average scores for questions three and four of the International Index of Erectile Function again were significantly higher for Viagra, compared with the placebo. The scores increased by 95 percent for question three and 140 percent for question four for those men who were on Viagra, versus only 10 percent and 13 percent, respectively, for those on placebo (please see Chapter 5 to review the IIEF questions). In this arm of the study, 74 percent of men reported improved erections on Viagra, versus only 19 percent on placebo.

As part of the questionnaire, efficacy of Viagra was also reviewed for five separate responses dealing with erectile-related activity, or so-called "domains of male sexual function." These included the areas of not only erectile function, but orgasmic function, sexual desire, intercourse satisfaction, and overall satisfaction. Figure 18 shows the clear results. It is important to note that the average scores for erectile function, orgasmic function, intercourse satisfaction, and overall satisfaction domains were higher with Viagra at the end of the study, compared with the placebo. Also, the scores increased in these categories from baseline to the end of the study for patients on Viagra, but not for patients on a placebo. Clearly, the men in this study benefited not only from a better erection, but also from improved sexual functioning associated with a better erection; in other words, a better orgasmic function, improved intercourse satisfaction, and overall satisfaction with sexual activity. Here we should also point out that there was no increase in sexual desire, but that is not surprising. In fact, by now we expect that. Remember, Viagra increases the penile response to sexual stimulation, but the drug Viagra itself is not a sexual stimulant. As such, its use alone cannot trigger sexual arousal. For sexual arousal to occur, visual, tactile, auditory, imaginative stimuli, or other "sensory" stimuli are needed.

Patients also kept an event-log in this study. During the last four weeks of the trial, 69 percent of all attempts to have sexual intercourse were successful in those men taking Viagra, compared with only 22 percent of men on a placebo. Furthermore, the number of successful attempts at sexual intercourse per month were higher among men receiving Viagra (5.9) than those receiving a placebo (1.5), and this was highly statistically significant (see Figure 19). Lastly, the side effects reported in this study were similar to side effects reported in other studies with Viagra. Headache, flushing, and dyspepsia (indigestion) were the most common and occurred in 6 percent to 18 percent of men in the dose-escalation study.

The overall conclusion of the authors of the study was that Viagra is an effective, well tolerated oral treatment for E.D.

Keeping Viagra in Perspective: In many instances, when results of a study involving a new drug are published, the medical journal will invite another expert to write an editorial, published in the same issue, to comment on different aspects of the findings. In this case, a leading urologist prepared the editorial, pointing out that the average scores for key questions regarding strength and maintenance of erections while on Viagra

Figure 19. Average scores for five IIEF questions

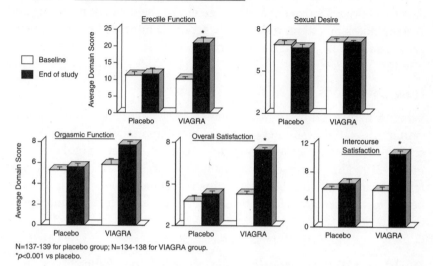

N=137-139 for placebo group; N=134-138 for VIAGRA group.
*$p<0.001$ vs placebo.

were not as high as for normal men; some men still were not able to achieve intercourse, despite the use of Viagra. Of course, no medicine is perfect, and it would be unrealistic to think that absolutely every man with E.D. who takes Viagra will benefit from the drug. Still, Viagra was very effective, and even the editorial points out that Viagra was effective in patients with organic, psychogenic, or mixed E.D. In this commentary, the author also compared the use of Viagra with the drug alprostadil. Alprostadil, or synthetic prostaglandin E_1, can be given by injection into the penis, and more recently, this drug may also be delivered via a suppository inserted into the urethra. This medication relaxes smooth muscle directly but must be given by local injection or into the urethra, which is awkward and may be painful. Alprostadil can also result in erections without sexual arousal, while Viagra requires sexual arousal in order to work.

The editorial also noted that since Viagra is known to be a safe and effective oral agent for E.D., it is likely that many more men will come forward and seek help for this condition.

Although the "Viagra-craze" is ongoing, it is reassuring to know that the use of this drug is based on a sound, scientifically based group of studies—not just anecdotes or word-of-mouth!

So, is Viagra effective? Suffice it to say that the information we have to date shows that 74 percent and 82 percent of the men taking 50 mg and 100 mg doses of Viagra, respectively, reported improved erections—improved sufficiently enough to experience satisfactory sexual intercourse.

How Long Does Viagra Take to Work?

When a man swallows a Viagra tablet, it is rapidly absorbed into his system; thus, the desired effect—to achieve an erection satisfactory for sexual intercourse—generally occurs in one hour after an oral dose (see Figure 20). The pharmaceutical manufacturer, Pfizer Inc, recommends taking Viagra one hour before anticipated sexual activity, but it can also be taken anywhere from four hours to approximately thirty minutes prior to sexual activity.

How Long Will an Erection Last after Taking Viagra?

Results of several studies show that taking one tablet of Viagra increased a man's ability to have an erection for up to two to four hours. In one study, the erections lasted eight to eleven minutes at the 50 mg dose, with sexual stimulation.

How Much Viagra Should You Take?

To answer this question, let your physician or health care professional be your guide. Once your physician has determined that you are suffering from E.D., your physician may want to look at possible causes, such as high blood pressure or diabetes, or he or she may simply decide to proceed to treatment with Viagra. To begin, the doctor will probably start you off on a dose of one 50 mg tablet about one hour before sexual activity. Depending on its effectiveness and tolerability, your physician may subsequently suggest increasing the dose up to a maximum of one 100 mg tablet or decreasing it to one 25 mg pill. To date, the current maximum recommended dosing frequency is once daily (see Figure 21).

Your physician may also suggest starting at the lower dose of Viagra—25 mg—if you have one or more of the following conditions: you are older than sixty-five, you have liver disease or severe kidney disease, or you are simultaneously using certain other drugs, including certain antibiotics and anti-ulcer medications. Also, while there isn't any reason

Figure 20. <u>VIAGRA generally should be taken approximately one hour before engaging in sexual activity</u>

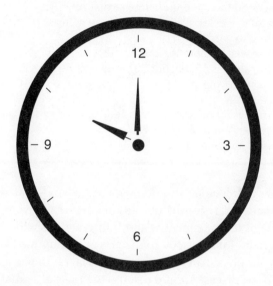

why you can't take Viagra with food, food can occasionally delay the rate of absorption of a drug, thereby slowing slightly the drug's onset of action. Do keep in mind that it is probably not a good idea to engage in sexual activity immediately after a heavy meal anyway, especially if you have a history of other medical problems such as heart disease.

Finally, there have been a few anecdotal reports of men who start on one dose of the drug, but on first usage they find the drug is not effective. With subsequent use, however, the drug works. Why? It's possible that initial "performance anxiety" occurs when a man attempts to have sexual intercourse after a long absence of sexual activity.

What You Need to Know to Take Viagra Safely and Effectively

As a reminder, men with E.D. should be evaluated by their physicians prior to receiving Viagra. As discussed earlier, the evaluation should include a thorough history and physical examination, as well as laboratory tests if your doctor determines they are needed. Underlying causes of

STEPS TO APPROPRIATE USE OF VIAGRA

1. Do *not* take Viagra if you are on nitrates.
2. Take Viagra orally one hour before sexual activity.
3. A fatty meal will delay absorption and may increase the time necessary for the drug to work.
4. Do not take Viagra more than once a day.
5. The starting dose is 50 mg, but if this does not work, discuss changing the dosage with your physician, increasing up to the 100 mg dose.
6. The most common side effects are headache, flushing, dyspepsia (indigestion), nasal congestion, transient blue-tinge in vision, and increased perception of brightness.
7. Viagra is *not* an aphrodisiac.

E.D., as well as risk factors, should be identified and treated as part of an overall treatment strategy—before any medicine is given. Most importantly, because of recent concerns about interactions with other drugs—especially nitrates—it is crucial to discuss any other medication you are taking with your physician *before* you take Viagra. In particular, patients with known heart disease should discuss the risks of sexual activity with their physician.

What Are the Side Effects?

To begin with, virtually every drug carries some side effects, even if they are very mild and transient. Viagra does indeed have side effects but fortunately, in most men these side effects are mild. In fact, studies showed that the rate of discontinuation due to side effects was only 2.5 percent for Viagra, not very different from the placebo, at 2.3 percent (see Figure 22). In general, side effects due to Viagra are both short-lived and mild-to-moderate. In one study in which 734 men received Viagra, the most common side effects reported were headaches, which 16 percent of the men experienced, followed by facial flushing (10 percent), dyspepsia or indigestion (7 percent), nasal congestion (4 percent), urinary tract infection (3 percent), and abnormal vision (3 percent). The abnormal vision was mild and transient and was primarily reported as a blue color-tinge to the vision, increased sensitivity to light, or blurred vision. At various medical meetings, medical investigators have reported the results of ophthalmologic testing that showed that some patients experi-

Figure 21. <u>Viagra is available in three doses</u>

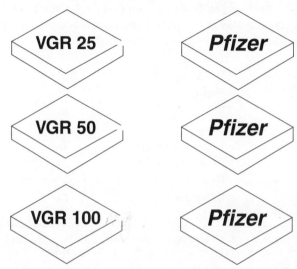

VIAGRA currently is available in three different doses: a 25-mg tablet, a 50-mg tablet, and a 100-mg tablet. The 50-mg dose is the most commonly prescribed dose. The diamond-shaped blue tablet is clearly marked with the dose on one side and the manufacturer identification on the other side, Pfizer.

enced a transient change in their ability to distinguish blue-green color vision, but there was no change in visual acuity, contrast sensitivity, visual fields, intraocular pressure, or other visual problems. (Table 13 lists side effects that may occur.) At the 100 mg dose of Viagra, dyspepsia and abnormal vision were more common than at lower doses. Finally, diarrhea, dizziness, and rash were seen in 3 percent, 2 percent, and 2 percent of men, respectively.

Importantly, priapism—a painful erection that endures for hours—a complication that has been reported with other therapies for E.D., is extremely rare with Viagra and causation remains to be determined. Finally, Viagra does not appear to affect sperm count or function.

Drug-Drug Interactions

By now, most of us recognize that it is inadvisable to take any prescription drug without informing our physician about any other drugs that we may be taking, including over-the-counter medications such as aspirin, cough-cold medications, antihistamines, and so forth. The reason

Table 13

The side effects of Viagra as reported in the prescribing information for Viagra (reported in ≥ 2 percent of patients and more frequent than placebo).*

Headache	16%
Flushing	10%
Dyspepsia	7%
Nasal Congestion	4%
Urinary tract infection	3%
Abnormal vision	3%
Diarrhea	3%
Dizziness	2%
Rash	2%

*These data were reported as of March, 1998. There could be other side effects/adverse effects that do not manifest until the drug has been on the market for some time.

Figure 22. VIAGRA: Discontinuation rate due to adverse events

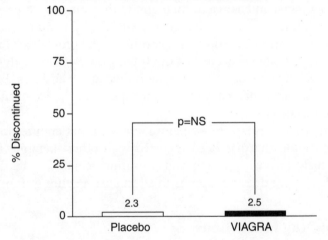

for this is clear: one drug may interact with another drug unfavorably, causing side effects that can range from a benign, transient mild headache to a far more severe reaction, such as life-threatening cardiac arrhythmia. Recently, for example, a very commonly prescribed antihistamine used to control allergy symptoms, Seldane®, was found to have a dangerous—and potentially fatal—effect if taken simultaneously with any number of commonly used antibiotics such as erythromycin. In very little time the U.S. Food and Drug Administration instructed the manufacturer to add a "black box" warning to prescribing information for Seldane®. (The package insert, or "PI," as it is usually known, provides the health care professional with all of the information necessary to prescribe the drug safely and appropriately.) A "black box" warning is so named because the important information outlined in heavy black lines alerts the physician and provides warning that the information contained therein is of a very serious nature. For Viagra, there is a serious and potentially life-threatening known drug-drug interaction: Viagra and *any* nitrate medication. Because of the serious nature of this drug-drug interaction, Viagra is *clearly* contraindicated in *all* patients taking nitrates (see "Contraindications to Taking Viagra" in this chapter). In addition, your physician may consider reducing your dose of Viagra if you are also taking a medication that is known to prolong Viagra's half-life. Such medications include, but are not limited to, the common antibiotic erythromycin, cimetidine (a common treatment for ulcers), and certain antifungal agents. Your doctor may also reduce your dose of Viagra if you have liver or kidney disease.

Precautions

Most drugs list one or more precautions associated with their use. This does not mean that the drug cannot be used, but simply that the drug should be used with caution in certain settings. For example, Viagra should be used cautiously in men with certain anatomical deformations of the penis, including Peyronie's disease, or in men who have conditions that predispose them to priapism. Some conditions that predispose to priapism include sickle cell anemia, leukemia, and multiple myeloma. It should also be given with caution in men with blood clotting problems, since there is no safety data available in these patients. Lastly, a drug used in treating acutely ill heart patients, sodium nitroprusside, seems to interact with Viagra to make blood platelets less likely to clot.

VIAGRA AND NITRATES

If your doctor tells you that your blood pressure is 130/80 mm Hg, what does it mean? Blood pressure is measured in terms of two factors: the systolic and the diastolic pressures in the arterial system. Thus, a reading of 130/80 mm Hg tells you the systolic and diastolic pressures, respectively. The number of millimeters a column of mercury rises as a result of the pressure is indicated by mm Hg.

Quite simply, *systolic* pressure is the maximum pressure put on the arterial system, and occurs during systole—that is, when the heart is pumping and sending blood through the arteries. Conversely, *diastolic* pressure indicates minimum pressure—that is, when the heart is resting between beats. This period in the cardiovascular cycle is diastole.

Results of clinical trials using Viagra showed that even healthy young men with no history of heart disease who took one sublingual nitroglycerin tablet—after ingesting one Viagra tablet—experienced a drop in systolic blood pressure of 25 to 51 mm Hg, along with a 26 mm Hg drop in diastolic pressure.

The bottom line? If you are taking nitrates for angina, and have a blood pressure of 130/90 mm Hg, taking just one Viagra tablet could trigger your blood pressure to drop well below a safe, healthy level; in fact, your blood pressure could suddenly fall to as low as 80/65 mm Hg! That's a long way from a normal reading of 120/80 mm Hg. So, if you're thinking about taking even *one* Viagra tablet while you also take nitrates—*don't do it!*

Thus, Viagra should be given with caution in patients who are also taking sodium nitroprusside. Finally, whether or not Viagra is safe in patients with a genetic disorder of the eye, retinitis pigmentosa, which may include an abnormality in the phosphodiesterase in the retina, is not known; thus, Viagra must be used with caution in these patients.

The effect of combining Viagra with other therapies for E.D. is also unknown; as such, these combinations are not recommended. Also, at the time of this writing Viagra was not yet FDA approved for women; therefore, women should not take it. There are no studies available on the effects of Viagra in pregnant women.

As discussed earlier, we know that men with E.D. are more likely to have risk factors for heart disease. Since there is a degree of cardiac risk associated with sexual activity, patients with heart disease should discuss sexual activity and therapies for E.D. with their physicians. (Please see "Can Having Sex Cause a Heart Attack?" in this chapter.) Lastly, other side effects due to Viagra may not become apparent until the drug is on the market for a longer period of time.

Contraindications to Taking Viagra

There is one major contraindication to taking Viagra that warrants your full, undivided attention: the use of nitrates. If you are taking organic nitrate drugs that are primarily used to treat angina pectoris, then you *cannot* take Viagra. Fortunately, recent data from the Massachusetts Male Aging Study suggested that only 4.6 percent of men with E.D. took nitrates for angina. Still, at the time of this writing, Viagra manufacturer Pfizer Inc has stated that this is an absolute contraindication. Why? You may recall that when we discussed the mechanisms of erection, we mentioned a substance called NO, or nitric oxide. Normally, there are always low levels of circulating NO throughout your circulatory system. Viagra enhances the vasodilator effect of NO; that is, NO acts to dilate or open up the arterioles, the smallest arteries, by inhibiting the effect of cGMP. In many men, Viagra induces a very mild reduction in blood pressure—about 8.4 mm Hg drop in systolic blood pressure, and a 5.5 mm Hg drop in diastolic pressure—and, in most men, this modest drop in blood pressure does not cause any symptoms, except the occasional mild headache and/or facial flushing. However, when a patient takes nitrates, the levels of NO in the circulation increase. Viagra then enhances, or potentiates, the vasodilatory effect of this higher level of NO, thereby causing a greater drop in blood pressure. This drop in blood pressure, associated with the use of nitrates plus Viagra, can be dramatic, even in men who are otherwise young and healthy. Unfortunately, the consequences of a major drop in blood pressure can be life-threatening. Symptoms of this sudden drop in blood pressure include dizziness, fainting, rapid heart beat, and loss of consciousness. If a man has underlying coronary heart disease or cerebrovascular disease, the possibility of a myocardial infarction (heart attack), stroke, or even death exists.

To learn more about the interactions of nitrates with Viagra, a study was designed involving healthy young men. These men, ages eighteen to forty-five, took a sublingual nitroglycerin tablet after taking Viagra. Most of them experienced a drop in systolic blood pressure by at least 25 mm Hg; in fact, some men experienced a drop in blood pressure of up to 51 mm Hg in systolic pressure and a 26 mm Hg drop in diastolic pressure. In other words, in a healthy young man, thirty years old, who has normal blood pressure of 120/80 mm Hg (the systolic and diastolic readings, respectively), the combination of Viagra and a sublingual nitroglycerin tablet can lead to a sudden drop in blood pressure—to 95/54 mm Hg! Overall, half of these healthy men experienced severe headaches, nausea, and dizziness, all the result of a sudden drop in blood pressure to too-low levels.

The most commonly used organic nitrates include sublingual nitroglycerin tablets as well as isosorbide dinitrate (Isordil®), isosorbide mononitrate (Imdur® and Ismo®), nitroglycerin patches, nitroglycerin paste, and a host of other formulations (see Table 14). If you have a history of angina pectoris and take nitrates, you must discuss this with your physician. Also, it's *very* important to remember that if your cardiologist or family physician has given you nitroglycerin or other nitrates to control your anginal pain—and you then go on to see a *different* physician to discuss your E.D.—you *must* tell that physician that you are on nitroglycerin or other nitrates. Remember, there are other therapies for E.D. besides Viagra and with patients on nitrates, these other therapies must be considered. If you take Viagra, develop chest pain, then go to an emergency room, you *must* tell the staff and attending physicians that you have taken Viagra. Otherwise, they could give you a nitrate medication to relieve chest pain, and nitrates and Viagra may *not* be used together. These drug interactions could be fatal.

But what if a man with angina discontinues his nitrate therapy in order to take Viagra? Frankly, this is a bad idea! A patient who has angina, discontinues his nitrates, and then takes Viagra may be able to engage in sexual activity, but it is also possible that an episode of angina (chest pain) could occur during sex. A patient who is accustomed to the quick relief from anginal pain that a sublingual nitroglycerin tablet can provide may reach for a tablet, only to discover that this drug-drug combination can cause very serious problems—even death. To date, in fact, nitrates are the only known drug-drug interaction with Viagra that led to a contraindication on the package insert (see "Viagra and Nitrates" in this chapter). As of this writing, sixty-nine verified deaths—out of approximately 2.5 million men on Viagra—have been reported after four months on the market. Of the 69 deaths in the United States, the men ranged in age from 29 to 87 years. Overall, 46 had documented cardiovascular events, including heart attacks and cardiac arrest. The average

Table 14

COMMONLY PRESCRIBED NITRATES

The following is a selected list of commonly prescribed nitrates by class from *Drug Facts and Comparisons*. Please consult your physician if you are using any of these medications, as they are contraindicated with the use of Viagra.

Nitrogylcerin	**Isosorbide mononitrate**
Deponit	Imdur
Minitran	ISMO
Nitrek	Isosorbide mononitrate
Nitro-Bid	Monoket
Nitro-Derm	**Isosorbide dinitrate**
Nitro-Dur	Dilatrate-SR
Nitrogard	Iso-bid
Nitroglycerin	Isordil
Nitroglycerine T/R	Isordil Tembids
Nitroglyn	Isosorbide Dinitrate
Nitrol Ointment	Isosorbide Dinitrate LA
Nitrolan	Sorbitrate
Nitrolingual Spray	Sorbitrate SA
Nitrong	**Pentaerythritol tetranitrate**
Nitropar	Peritrate
Nitropress	Peritrate SA
Nitro SA	**Erythrityl tetranitrate**
Nitrostat	Cardilate
Nitrospan	**Isosorbide dinitrate/phenobarbitol**
Nitro-Trans System	Nitro Transdermal
Isordil with PB	
Nitro-Time	
Transderm-Nitro	
Tridil	

Amyl Nitrite or Amyl Nitrate: This formulation is sometimes abused and is known by various names, such as "poppers."

Figure 23. VIAGRA Efficacy: ED patients with depression (improvement in erections)

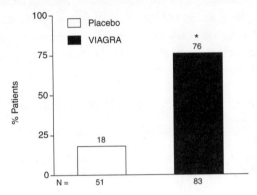

*p<0.0001 vs placebo.

Reprinted with permission from Viagra (sildemafil citrate) Tablets, Product Monograph. ©1998 Pfizer Inc.

age (in 55 patients where age was reported) was 64 years. Twelve of these men had self-medicated or were given nitroglycerin or a nitrate medication—a clear contraindication with the use of Viagra. In addition, it is now known that 25 of the 69 patients died or had symptoms leading to death within 4 to 5 hours of using Viagra. It has also been established that 51 of the 69 men had one or more risk factors for heart disease (i.e., cigarette smoking, high blood pressure, elevated LDL cholesterol level, diabetes, etc.) present. Three other men with no known history of cardiovascular disease or risk factors were shown to have severe coronary artery disease at autopsy.

Sexual Activity, Heart Disease, and Viagra

It is important to note that on August 10, 1998, the American College of Cardiology (ACC) in conjunction with the American Heart Association (AHA) issued a brief commentary, called "Summary Statement on the Use of Sildenafil (Viagra) in Patients at Clinical Risk from Cardiovascular Effects." This document is still evolving, and currently the ACC and AHA plan to release their formal statement in December 1998. However, in light of the intense interest in Viagra—coupled with the 69 deaths of men in the U.S. using Viagra reported through July 1998—the ACC and

Figure 24. VIAGRA efficacy: ED patients with spinal cord injury (ability to maintain an erection)

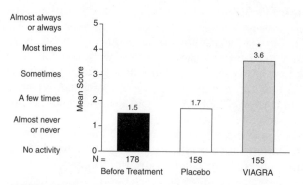

*p<0.0001 vs placebo.

Patients completed the IIEF, a sexual function questionnaire to evaluate the major effiacy variables, the ability of the patient to achieve and maintain erections sufficient for intercourse.

Reprinted with permission from Viagra (sildemafil citrate) Tablets, Product Monograph. ©1998 Pfizer Inc.

AHA decided to issue "interim recommendations," to help physicians manage their cardiac patients on Viagra. To summarize, these interim guidelines state:

- Viagra is absolutely contraindicated in patients on chronic nitrate therapy; those who use short-acting nitrate medication; and in those who inhale nitrates, such as amyl nitrates or "poppers."

In addition, the ACC and AHA recommendations point out that the cardiovascular effects of Viagra may be potentially hazardous in certain patients; thus, doctors must exercise caution when treating the following patients:

- Patients with active coronary ischemia (low coronary blood flow) who are not on nitrates
- Patients with congestive heart failure and borderline low blood pressure and borderline low volume status
- Patients on a complicated multi-drug, antihypertensive program
- Patients on drugs (e.g., erythromycin, cimetidine) or who have conditions (e.g., liver or renal disease) that can prolong the half-life of Viagra.

SOME CARDIOVASCULAR STATISTICS TO CONSIDER

Within the first four months of Viagra being on the market, sixty-nine verified deaths were reported in the U.S. out of approximately 2.5 million men. Overall, forty-six had cardiovascular events; twenty-one were heart attacks and seventeen were cardiac arrests. Twelve cases involved nitrates. We already know that Viagra is contraindicated for use with nitrates. The FDA reviewed this data and at present the FDA has not recommended any changes in labeling. The FDA also said that they would continue to monitor post-marketing safety.

How do sixty-nine cardiac deaths out of 2.5 million men nationwide during approximately four months stack up against other data? Is this a major medical concern? For comparison, our research group recently had the chance to review coronary deaths in Los Angeles County (a population of about 8.8 million people). Every *day* in this county alone there are an average of seventy-three deaths due to coronary artery disease. Furthermore, statistics from the National Center for Health Statistics show that the underlying rate of death from all causes in men over forty-five is almost 1,600 deaths per million per month. The American Heart Association estimates that, in men, the monthly total number of deaths due to cardiovascular disease is 185 to 275 out of one million. Of note, over 80 percent of prescriptions for Viagra have been for men over the age of fifty. Remember, coronary artery disease is the leading cause of death of mankind. Thus, sixty-nine deaths among men who were mainly older (the average age was sixty-four years) out of a population of 2.5 million, over a four-month period of time, did not cause undue concern within the FDA.

—ROBERT A. KLONER, M.D., PH.D.

Clearly, it is mandatory for you to consult your physician before taking *any* prescription medication, including Viagra. The risk of sexual activity and taking Viagra should be discussed with your physician.

As you now know, many of the same risk factors for coronary artery disease are also risk factors for E.D. We discussed these risk factors in Chapter 2, but it's worth reviewing here, too. These risk factors include abnormalities in blood cholesterol level, diabetes, smoking, high blood pressure, and aging.

Hypertension: Men with high blood pressure do respond well to Viagra. For example, results of clinical studies show that 68 percent of men with hypertension reported improvement in their erections on Viagra. In

Pfizer's reported studies, Viagra was added to several usual antihypertension medicines and caused only small decreases in blood pressure, similar to patients not taking antihypertensive agents.

Coronary Heart Disease and Risk of Death: There is always some (although usually small) risk of having a cardiac event, including a heart attack and death, with sexual activity. Since E.D. is fairly common in patients with heart disease, patients with E.D. should discuss sexual activity with their physicians before trying Viagra. Clearly, patients who have coronary artery disease with angina and are taking nitroglycerin *cannot* take Viagra. However, in patients with coronary heart disease without angina, an exercise tolerance test—usually performed on a treadmill—may provide the patient and physician with useful information to reach an informed decision regarding the cardiovascular safety of sexual activity.

Overall, sixty-nine men in the United States out of 2.5 million men taking Viagra have died by the end of July, 1998. Fifty-one of them had risk factors for heart disease. Early on, the FDA released a statement suggesting that these events did not indicate newly identified problems with Viagra. It is likely that other than the cases associated with concomitant use of nitrates, the risk of a heart attack with sexual activity—which is a known risk—contributed. (See "Some Cardiovascular Statistics to Consider" in this chapter.)

Diabetes: Men with diabetes also fare well on Viagra. Specifically, the results of one double-blind, twelve-week study showed that improvement in erections occurred in 57 percent of diabetic men receiving Viagra, compared with 10 percent who took a placebo.

As we discussed in Chapter 5, patients with E.D. should be evaluated by their physicians prior to receiving Viagra. The physician's evaluation should include a thorough history and physical examination, and laboratory tests if indicated. Underlying causes and risk factors should be identified and treated as part of an overall treatment strategy—before any medicine is given.

Does Viagra Work in Depressed Men? To determine whether or not Viagra would be effective in clinically depressed men, medical investigators reviewed the results of nine double-blind, placebo-controlled studies, conducted from six weeks up to six months. At the end \of the studies, 76 percent of men reported that they had improved erections (see Figure

MORE CONCERN ABOUT THE NITRATE-VIAGRA INTERACTION

As of the end of July, 1998, Viagra had been on the market in the U.S. for approximately four months; it is currently estimated that about 2.5 million U.S. men were on the medication. In August, the FDA released information stating that sixty-nine confirmed deaths had been reported in the U.S. Twelve of these deaths involved the use of nitrates. Pfizer had urged physicians to adhere to the warning *not* to give Viagra to patients taking nitrates in any form. As we discussed earlier, the nitrate-Viagra combination can be deadly. Middle-aged men with E.D. are likely to have other risk factors for coronary artery disease; it is known that sexual activity is associated with a small but significant risk of having a heart attack, or a cardiac arrhythmia (an irregular heart rhythm), which can be associated with a heart attack or even death. As such, it is possible that some of these deaths might have occurred even without the use of Viagra, especially when one considers that at least 2.5 million men are on this drug. Nevertheless, these deaths are obviously a concern, so we are repeating the importance of *not* taking Viagra if you are on nitrates. In fact, in response to earlier deaths, Dr. Ivy Kopec of the FDA said that the "U.S. FDA continues to believe the drug is safe and effective for its labeled indication and intended patient population." The FDA requested that Pfizer provide men receiving the drug with more information on the proper use of the drug.

It is our understanding that Pfizer has sent notices to emergency room personnel (ERs) to ask patients admitted to the emergency rooms with chest pain, whether during or after sexual activity, if they have taken Viagra. Of course, if you don't inform the ER physician, he or she may give you a nitrate—most commonly sublingual nitroglycerin—and this will put you at serious risk of a major drop in blood pressure. Again, the nitrate-Viagra interaction is *very serious* business.

---

23). Fortunately, there are not only highly effective and safe treatments available today for depression, but now there also is a highly effective and safe oral medication for E.D.

What About Spinal Cord Injury? Frankly, it is likely that many men who have sustained a spinal cord injury may, in fact, view Viagra as a panacea. In one group of men with spinal cord injury, of whom 137 out of 178 had severe spinal cord lesions according to classifications established by the American Spinal Injury Association (ASIA), an amazing 80 percent of patients reported improvement in their ability to have sexual intercourse (see Figure 24).

Surgeries: Two surgical procedures in particular are also associated with E.D.: TURP, or transurethral resection of the prostate, and radical prostatectomy. Again, in both of these clinical settings, results of studies demonstrated that Viagra is clearly effective in improving erections in many of these patients. Specifically, data obtained from eight double-blind, placebo-controlled studies, carried out over six weeks to six months, showed that at the end of the studies, 61 percent of TURP patients said their erections were improved, whereas, in the group of men who had undergone a radical prostatectomy, 43 percent reported Viagra was effective in improving their erections. These findings indicate that Viagra is useful for some men who have had these types of surgeries.

So You're Getting Older! Let's consider simple aging first, since more and more baby-boomers are passing the great divide: age fifty. Although we qualify for our AARP (American Association of Retired Persons) card on our fiftieth birthday, today the term "elderly" usually refers to those sixty-five years of age and older. In studies, these men had a rate of erectile improvement with Viagra of 67 percent—close to the 75 percent rate of improvement seen in younger patients!

Will Viagra Work in Every Man with E.D.?

To date, the statistics look like this: at the 50 mg or 100 mg dose, Viagra is effective in 74 percent to 82 percent of men with E.D. Specifically, Viagra is effective in all of the conditions discussed here (organic and pyschogenic causes of E.D.), although the degree of efficacy may not be the same or as great as in uncomplicated E.D., depending upon the underlying cause of the E.D. Still, Viagra seems to work equally well in older versus younger patients, in patients with high blood pressure, in patients taking high blood pressure medications, and in depressed patients. The response to Viagra is better than a placebo in other serious conditions too, such as diabetes, spinal cord injury, TURP, and radical prostatectomy.

And what about normal men who don't have E.D.? To date, no controlled studies have been carried out to evaluate the effects of Viagra in men who don't have E.D. Here, it's important to point out Viagra is a *prescription* medication with a specific indication: E.D. Thus, it should only be used as indicated.

Sexually Transmitted Diseases: Finally, Viagra offers no protection against sexually transmitted diseases such as human immunodeficiency virus (HIV). Therefore, it is important to consider protective measures—safe sex techniques—during sexual activity.

Other Therapies

Currently, there are six types of treatments for E.D. available today: counseling, oral medications, medicines delivered directly to the penis by either injection or insertion into the urethra, vacuum erection devices, vascular surgery, and penile prostheses.

Oral Medications: Other oral medications (pills) are available for the treatment of E.D. besides Viagra, but none of these have the same efficacy as Viagra. In the past, these medications were the only ones available, and the long-term satisfaction rate was less than 20 percent. Yohimbine (Yocon), for one, is a derivative from the bark of the Yohimbine tree, and it increases sex drive as well as, potentially, penile blood flow. Common side effects include headaches and high blood pressure. Another agent, isoxsuprine (Vasodilan®), is frequently used with men who are cigarette smokers; it is most effective when combined with smoking reduction. Vasodilan works by dilating blood vessels. Side effects are extremely rare, but it is contraindicated in men with severe heart disease.

Trazodone (Desyrel®) is another drug that is frequently used. This medication was first developed as a sleeping pill and antidepressant. However, men taking this medication reported an adverse side effect of priapism. Trazodone is now used to treat E.D., but patients should still be aware of this potential side effect as well as drowsiness. Trazodone appears to have its greatest effect early in the morning.

All of these medications must be taken daily. Unlike Viagra, they are not "on demand" medications. In addition, none of these medications are effective with the first pill and should be taken for at least one month to determine if they will be effective.

Oral Phentolamine (Vasomax™): This oral pill is currently under study for E.D. Called Vasomax, it is an oral form of the vasodilating agent phentolamine. Phentolamine is a drug which, in experimental studies, causes relaxation and dilation of the tissue in the corpus cavernosum. Phentola-

PATIENTS TAKING VIAGRA AT JOHNS HOPKINS: RESULTS

At our institution (Johns Hopkins), we treated a total of 298 men with Viagra during the first six weeks it was on the market. Follow-up information is now available on 267 of those men. Patients filled out both baseline and follow-up questionnaires to measure their erectile function, response to the medication, and presence of side effects. Overall, 72 percent of men reported satisfaction with Viagra therapy for erectile dysfunction with short-term follow-up. The response rate was directly proportional to baseline sexual function (*i.e.*, patients with better baseline function were more likely to respond to Viagra). However, many patients with minimal baseline erectile function had a good response to Viagra as reflected by the overall high response rate of 72 percent. We also observed significant variation in response to Viagra based upon medical illness.

Finally, side effects were relatively minor and uncommon. Headaches, facial flushing, and nasal congestion were the most common side effects, ranging from 9 to 15 percent of the patients. Vision disturbances were extremely rare at 2 percent. None of our patients stopped taking medication because of the side effects.

—JONATHAN P. JAROW, M.D.

mine was one of the agents that worked when it was injected with a needle directly into the penis. Often when injected in this fashion, it was given with other vasodilating agents (such as papaverine, and alprostadil).

Vasomax has a different mechanism of action than Viagra. It works by blocking a portion of the sympathetic nervous system known as alpha receptors, which cause constriction of blood vessels and, as such, it acts to dilate blood vessels and increase blood flow to the penis.

Pioneering work by several investigators has shown that giving phentolamine orally, or bucally (placed on strips and applied to the inner cheek), could produce full erections in patients with E.D. Soon thereafter, work began on developing an oral form of the drug. The pill form dissolves quickly, with levels in the bloodstream peaking after thirty minutes of ingestion. In a pilot study, patients with E.D. due to organic cause underwent a controlled study with oral phentolamine. While only two out of ten patients achieved full erection with placebo, five out of ten achieved full erection at the 40 mg dose, and four out of ten achieved it at the 60 mg dose.

Additional studies with larger numbers of patients conducted both in and outside of the United States suggested that men taking Vasomax had a 40 percent to 60 percent response rate. The optimal dose appeared to be 40 mg. In one study, men older than fifty had the best response rates, compared with younger men. Nasal stuffiness was reported as a side effect.

To date, the FDA has not yet approved Vasomax for the treatment of E.D. Whether Vasomax will work in patients who do not respond to Viagra, and whether Viagra will work in patients who do not respond to Vasomax, remains to be determined. Whether or not one will be able to use the two drugs together is also unknown at this time.

Apomorphine (Provim™). Apomorphine is currently under investigation as a possible oral treatment for E.D. It has been available since 1869 and has been used parenterally as an emetic agent and as an anti-Parkinsonian drug. It is a centrally acting dopamine agonist. Researchers have developed apomorphine as a sublingual formulation, and the agent is undergoing evaluation for the treatment of E.D.

It appears that apomorphine is ideal for oral treatment of E.D. It is rapidly absorbed, and effects are observed within twenty to forty-five minutes after administration in the presence of sexual stimulation. However, one of the side effects—considerable nausea—may make apomorphine an undesirable choice for treatment.

Constrictive Bands: These fancy rubber bands, or O-rings, have been used with a great deal of success in men who have no trouble achieving an erection, but difficulty maintaining it. The success rate in maintaining erections with constrictive bands is approximately 35 percent. This treatment option is inexpensive and safe, if the bands are kept on for less than thirty minutes at a time.

Vacuum Erection Device: This is a nonsurgical device that is safe, relatively inexpensive, and effective. The vacuum device is comprised of a plastic cylinder, pump, and tight rubber bands. The plastic cylinder is placed over the penis and pressed against the body to create an airtight seal. The hand pump is then used to create a vacuum within the cylinder. This vacuum draws blood into the penis, and the rubber bands are placed around the base of the penis to trap the blood within the penis. Overall, this device works in approximately 90 percent of men, but many men and their partners don't like it. The erection is hinged, since the erection does not extend beyond the rubber bands at the base of the penis. Moreover, the penis is cold to the touch since the rubber bands cut off circulation. In addition, approximately 40 percent of men experience significant discomfort associated with the use of these tight rubber bands. The device is available over-the-counter and costs between $200 and $300. Approximately 55 percent of men who try this device are satisfied with it.

Injections: The second most popular and effective medical therapy after oral medications is injection therapy. Various vasoactive medications produce an erection in men after injection directly into the erectile tissue of the penis. These medications include but are not limited to papaverine, prostaglandin E_1 and phentolamine, and may be used singly or in combination. The amount of drug injected determines the duration and strength of the erection. Every man requires a dose that can only be determined by trial and error, through test injections in the physician's office. A dose of a vasoactive agent that is too low, for example, will not be effective, while a dose that is too high will produce priapism. Generally, we aim for a dose that produces a full erection lasting approximately sixty to ninety minutes. Patients who are interested in injection therapy are taught how to perform the injections properly, and the proper dose is determined over a course of two to three office visits.

There are very few complications associated with injection therapy when performed properly, but the main complication is priapism. The

IF YOU DON'T THINK AN INJECTION INTO THE PENIS WORKS . . .

For centuries, there was little man could do to correct E.D. Many "potions" were tried, as we discussed in Chapter 1; still, there was generally little improvement. Then, over the past couple of decades, researchers began to come up with some medical approaches that were effective in some men, even if these alternatives (such as injections and surgery) seemed undesirable. In fact, just over fifteen years ago, a urologist at the annual scientific meeting of the American Urological Association who was working with vasodilating substances to determine their efficacy in treating E.D. decided to show the physician-audience just how effective an injection could be. During the course of his presentation, the doctor announced that he had injected a vasodilating substance directly into his penis approximately one hour before his talk. He stepped from around the podium, dropped his trousers, and literally showed the audience the effects of the injection; i.e., his erect penis. Suffice it to say that most in the audience have never forgotten it!

penis may be permanently damaged if an erection persists for longer than six hours. Other potential complications include bruising, infection, and scarring, but these complications should not occur if a proper technique is followed. These medications are available by prescription, and the cost ranges from $40 to $120 for a month's supply. The overall satisfaction rate for injection therapy is greater than 70 percent. Still, there is a high dropout rate for this therapy. Interestingly enough, approximately 40 percent of men who were initially happy using this therapy discontinued use within five years.

Suppositories: The same medication used for injection therapy—prostaglandin E$_1$—is now also available as a suppository, to be inserted in the urethra. This formulation is sold under the brand name, MUSE® (alprostadil). It removes the fear and discomfort associated with penile injections, but this also results in sacrificing efficacy—in fact, the long term efficacy of MUSE® is only about 20 percent. Side effects include pain, light-headedness and, rarely, prolonged erection. To begin, a test dose is given in the physician's office, to check for side effects and dosing before prescribing the medication. The cost of MUSE is relatively high, approximately $130 for five doses.

Vascular Surgery: Although vascular abnormalities are the most frequent physical cause of E.D., very few men with E.D. are candidates for vascular surgery. The presence of discrete blockage in the arteries supplying blood to the erectile bodies can be corrected by arterial bypass surgery, analogous to what is done for cardiac bypass surgery. Only young, healthy men who do not smoke are candidates for this procedure. In these patients, the success rate is approximately 80 percent, which means full restoration of sexual function. This is an expensive surgical procedure to perform, and requires hospitalization for about five days.

Venous ligation, another procedure, was once performed in men with evidence of venous leakage who had normal arterial blood flow. This procedure is no longer performed, except as an investigational procedure, because of a very poor success rate coupled with a high complication rate.

Penile implants: Surgical placement of a penile implant is the most successful long-term treatment for men with organic E.D. Both patient and partner satisfaction rate for this treatment option is greater than 90 percent. However, this option is usually reserved as a last resort because it requires surgery. Overall, there are many penile prostheses available, but they can be divided into two types: inflatable and semi-rigid.

Inflatable and Semi-Rigid Prostheses: The inflatable device is the most popular penile prothesis, but it has a higher complication rate than the semi-rigid prosthesis, which is satisfactory for most men. Neither the patient nor the partner can tell the difference between the two types of prostheses during sexual intercourse. The main difference between these two devices is evident when the patient is *not* having sex. The inflatable device assumes a more natural appearance when deflated, while the semi-rigid always remains semi-erect. Thin men who wear tight fitting clothes may be uncomfortable with a semi-rigid prosthesis. The cost of a penile prosthesis ranges from $10,000 to $15,000, and is covered by most health-insurance companies. This procedure is performed under anesthesia and requires overnight hospitalization. The main risk is infection, which occurs in 3 percent of men despite many efforts to prevent it. Mechanical failure can occur with any device, but is more common with the inflatable prosthesis. Overall, approximately 15 percent of the inflatable prosthetics will break within the first five years. An infected penile prosthesis has to be removed, whereas a broken one can be repaired or replaced. Because of the cost and risks associated with a penile prosthesis, this option is recommended only in patients who have failed or do not desire medical forms of therapy.

Counseling: Many couples would benefit from counseling even if the cause of the E.D. is physical, since sexual problems may frequently lead to problems in a couple's relationship, or vice versa. Counseling is the treatment of choice for men who have psychogenic E.D. or problems with premature ejaculation. However, medical therapies are sometimes used to help men get through a rough period in their lives. Sex therapists are specialized in dealing with these problems, but may not be available in all communities.

Does Viagra Help if You Don't Have E.D.?

In patients who have no trouble achieving erections with sexual stimulation, Viagra is unlikely to add anything. Viagra does not make a normal erection harder, nor will Viagra make an erection last longer.

CAN HAVING SEX CAUSE A HEART ATTACK?

There is a small but finite risk of having a cardiac event—such as a heart attack or stroke—during sexual activity. After all, sex is exercise and must be considered as such. Just as men with heart disease are at risk when they shovel snow, so too should they be careful when engaging in sexual activity. It is likely, then, that some of the men who died and were taking Viagra did so because of this risk. In fact, it is most likely for a heart attack to occur in patients with risk factors for coronary artery disease (such as smoking, hypertension, high cholesterol, and so on)—the very same risk factors associated with E.D. However, again, the risk is small.

In 1996, James Muller, M.D. and his coworkers published a significant study on this subject in the *Journal of the American Medical Association*. They looked at 858 sexually active patients who had experienced heart attacks and analyzed potential triggers of heart attacks immediately prior to the event. Of these 858 patients, only twenty-seven (3 percent) reported sexual activity within two hours prior to the attack. The authors calculated that sexual activity contributed to the onset of a heart attack in only 0.9 percent of cases and that the absolute hourly risk of sex increasing the chance of having a heart attack was only one chance in a million for a healthy individual. Surprisingly, risks of having a heart attack with sex were not increased in patients with prior histories of angina pectoris compared with patients without angina. Patients involved in routine exercise were less likely to have heart attacks due to sexual activity.

continued next page

How Does Viagra Affect Other Aspects of Male Sexuality?

In studies that utilized sexual function questionnaires in patients enrolled in Viagra trials, the medical researchers were able to obtain additional information. Specifically, the International Index of Erectile Function, or IIEF, questionnaire was used. Overall, patients with E.D. had low baseline scores for all aspects of sexual function measured. But, with the use of Viagra, the patients reported an increase in frequency, firmness, and maintenance of erections. Interestingly, the patients also reported an increase in "frequency of orgasm, frequency and level of desire; frequency, satisfaction, and enjoyment of intercourse; and overall relationship satisfaction." These findings are very good news indeed because they suggest that Viagra may result in a "spill-over" effect, whereby *continued from page 120*

What is the physiological cost to the heart during sexual activity? In general, it is modest. During sexual activity, there is a moderate, gradual increase in heart rate and blood pressure for periods of five to fifteen minutes. Heart rate tends to increase up to 120 to 130 beats per minute, and systolic blood pressure increases to 150 to 180 mm Hg. Patients with coronary artery disease or suspected coronary artery disease or patients with E.D. who have coronary risk factors should discuss the issue with their physician. The physician might order an exercise treadmill or bicycle test or other stress test that will help to determine the patient's exercise tolerance and whether the patient exhibits signs, symptoms, or electrocardiographic abnormalities consistent with coronary artery narrowing and low blood flow to areas of the heart. A radionuclide tracer might be injected intravenously, which will help to determine whether blood flow to the heart is adequate or compromised.

Sexual activity following a heart attack or coronary artery bypass usually can be resumed by most patients after about four to six weeks. This is, of course, best discussed with your physician. One general rule of thumb is that if a patient can climb two flights of stairs after such an event, then he or she may resume sexual activity. However, your physician may want to conduct an exercise test before giving you the go-ahead to attempt sexual activity. When sexual activity is resumed, it should be done in a quiet, comfortable setting when the patient is free of stress and is rested. Intercourse should be postponed for one to three hours after eating a full meal or after exercise. A familiar, comfortable sexual position should be used, and, of course, if you are taking nitrates in any form, Viagra is contraindicated.

other aspects of the sexual act are improved as a result of being able to maintain an erection.

• • •

Now let's revisit this chapter's title: Is Viagra a wonder drug? The answer is a resounding yes! There is no question that Viagra *is* a wonder drug. Viagra is the first oral FDA-approved drug that is effective in treating E.D. Overall, it works in 74 to 82 percent of patients at the 50 and 100 mg dose, respectively. The drug is easy to take, is taken only when needed, and has a very favorable side-effect profile. In addition, few would argue that this drug may have the ability to improve sexual relationships between partners. But remember: Viagra it is not an aphrodisiac, and like all drugs, Viagra has certain limitations. For example, Viagra does not work in about 20 percent of patients, its efficacy is less in diabetics, and in patients who have had prostate surgery. Finally, Viagra is contraindicated in patients who take organic nitrates.

8

You and Your Mate
How Viagra May Alter
the Sexual Landscape

At the time of this writing, Viagra has only been available in the United States for four months. To date, more than 3.6 million prescriptions have been filled, making it the fastest-selling prescription drug in the history of American medicine. It's still a bit too early to know how Viagra may change the sexual landscape in the long-term, but already many men are reporting changes in their relationships with their partners. Frankly, it remains to be seen whether our speculations will be born out, but we predict Viagra *will* change the sexual landscape—possibly to as great or even to a greater extent than the advent of the birth control pill in 1960.

The Positive Psychological Effects of Viagra in Men

Like it or not, having sex involves a certain degree of "performance," and men are expected to perform. If you can't perform or if you perform poorly, it's normal to feel uptight, and we all know that this usually leads to an even poorer performance. Thus, the vicious cycle begins. This "performance anxiety" is a significant problem, especially in men with E.D. A man who has E.D. and fails to perform may also experience depression. Then, the depression itself contributes to the cycle of E.D. E.D. begets anxiety and depression, and they, in turn, beget E.D. Viagra helps break the cycle; this medication makes an erection possible, so the performance anxiety associated with E.D. is reduced, and often, the depression associated with E.D. is also reduced. Men can then begin to feel more relaxed about sexual pleasure, and this, in turn, allows them and their partner to enjoy sexual activity to a greater extent.

"I feel like I'm twenty-five—okay, thirty, again!" With that enthusiastic endorsement, Mike L., a lively sixty-year-old who, by his own account, has had a terrific marriage and a sexually fulfilling relationship with his wife of thirty years, talked candidly about how he found his way to Dr. Jarow's office, and why he was willing—more than willing—to take Viagra. After years of sharing an emotionally intimate, and physically mutually rewarding relationship, Mike L. found himself "losing it," as he put it. The decline in his ability to achieve and sustain an erection sufficient for sexual intercourse took place over several months, and its effect on both Mike and his spouse was clear. "She wanted me to see a doctor in no time flat," Mike told us. He preferred to wait a bit, believing he'd bounce back. But it didn't happen. Then, Mike was referred to Dr. Jarow, a leading urologist in the Baltimore area where Mike lives. "The rest, as they say, is history," Mike said. "I'm back—no, *we're* back—to our old happy, functional selves, thanks to Viagra."

Viagra: A Fountain of Youth

Does Viagra make men feel younger? In a recent *Time* magazine article, Bob Guccione, the publisher of *Penthouse* magazine, said "the ability to have sex by older men will make them healthier and live longer. It will fool the biological clock when men are still active in later years. It is a very significant effect of the drug that many haven't contemplated." This statement is unsubstantiated. It's important for all men and women to appreciate that, from both a pharmacological and physiological standpoint, there is *no* evidence whatsoever in the medical literature to support the idea that Viagra is a "fountain of youth." Still, it is likely that some men, like a couple of those in Dr. Jarow's practice, may experience some sense of transient youthfulness with the drug.

One thing is for sure: due to the availability of Viagra, men who never sought treatment before for E.D. are now "coming out of the closet" in droves. Up until the introduction of Viagra, approximately 90 percent of men with E.D.—that's right, 90 percent—did *not* seek treatment for their condition. Many were simply too embarrassed, and frankly, most physicians rarely took a comprehensive sexual history from their patients, so E.D. usually went undetected. To date, Viagra has led to more than 2.5 million men seeking treatment, and in that process, some of these men are obtaining additional medical care for other conditions they didn't know they had, such as high blood pressure, elevated cholesterol, diabetes, and so forth. Today, health care professionals know that men who present with E.D. may easily have another medical condition that is causing the E.D. Thus, a visit to the doctor's office for E.D. can now result in getting treatment for other medical disorders. Early, effective treatment for hypertension and diabetes, to name a few, can help reduce hospitalizations—and may even help prolong life.

Viagra in Couples: The Positive Potential

Because Viagra is safe and so effective in so many different men—younger and older, men with concomitant diseases, men on various medications, and so on—it is likely to be used by millions and millions of men. Since Viagra allows more men to achieve and maintain an erection adequate for sexual intercourse, intimacy between couples is likely to be restored—maybe even enhanced. Of course, the sexual desire has to be there to begin with. Remember, Viagra is *not* an aphrodisiac; it only enhances a man's ability to have an erection, provided he is sexually stimulated. Still, many couples who would like to resume normal sexual relations, but have faltered due to E.D., will now be able to experience what is probably the greatest physical pleasure that two individuals can share.

Bill K., a fifty-six-year-old professional who is one of Dr. Jarow's patients, now takes Viagra. He says he feels like life has never treated him better. After a few years of a declining sex life—something that distressed Bill and his wife terribly—he decided to seek treatment in early 1998 (see Figure 25). Understanding that FDA approval of Viagra was just around the corner (it was approved in late March 1998), Bill decided to wait in order to try this new, oral medication. "I've never looked back!" he said. "I'm grateful to the scientists, the researchers, all of the people who must have worked on this to help make it possible. You know," he added," it got to the point where my wife and I were actually altering our evening routines a bit—anything to avoid our traditional 'signals' to 'let's make love,' because both of us ultimately became too concerned that I just couldn't perform. Viagra's changed all that. Now, I just don't worry about what's going to happen . . . if it looks like we'll feel like having

**Figure 25. The downward spiral of ED:
how his dysfunction affects both of you**

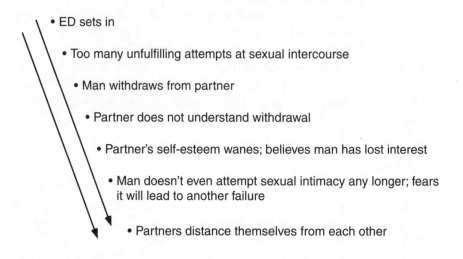

• ED sets in

• Too many unfulfilling attempts at sexual intercourse

• Man withdraws from partner

• Partner does not understand withdrawal

• Partner's self-esteem wanes; believes man has lost interest

• Man doesn't even attempt sexual intimacy any longer; fears it will lead to another failure

• Partners distance themselves from each other

sex, I take a Viagra, nature takes its course, and both of us have never felt more relieved—and happier!" (see Figure 26.)

This man's description of how the use of Viagra enabled him and his wife to renew sexual intimacy also conveys a subtle but *key* point about this medication; namely, that E.D. doesn't just affect a man, it affects a partner *and* the relationship, too. Although E.D. is generally not triggered by a problem in the relationship, it can—and sadly, often does—lead to problems between partners, especially when the couple doesn't understand the causes of E.D.

Viagra may well bring many of these couples together, and this renewed union could ultimately even strengthen the family. Interestingly enough, Pfizer Inc, the manufacturer of Viagra, even went so far as to contact Vatican officials before the drug was made available. Why? Because part of the teachings of the Catholic church foster conjugal relations, especially to procreate. In fact, in Roman Catholicism, impotency has always been one of the very, very few reasons that the Church would sanction an annulment, or dissolution, of the marriage. On the other hand, if you and your partner are having other difficulties, it is highly *unlikely* that Viagra will play any role in turning your relationship around.

Figure 26. The upward spiral of VIAGRA: how this drug affects both of you

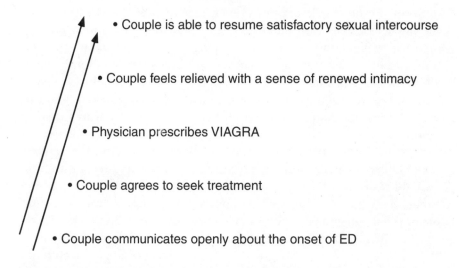

• Couple is able to resume satisfactory sexual intercourse

• Couple feels relieved with a sense of renewed intimacy

• Physician prescribes VIAGRA

• Couple agrees to seek treatment

• Couple communicates openly about the onset of ED

Viagra in Couples: What's the Downside?

While the hope is that men with E.D. who are treated with Viagra will respond favorably, thereby possibly improving their relationships and bringing the couples closer together, one could also ask: could the opposite occur? For example, is it possible that an older man, one who has been faithful to his wife, may now feel a renewed sense of vigor and potency, and suddenly find that his eye is now far more easily captured by other women? There already have been such cases reported; only time will tell whether or not a scenario like this one will become common. Clearly, no medication is responsible for the choice of sexual partners. A more subtle effect on the relationship, we think, is likely to go as follows: after several years of E.D., couples—especially older couples—settle into acceptance patterns. They may now be accustomed to not having sexual intercourse and have found other pathways to maintain emotional intimacy. Now, with Viagra, the man may experience a highly renewed interest in activating their sexual relationship again, whereas his wife has more or less lost interest. Of course, the opposite can also occur; i.e., a woman can "pressure" her mate into getting Viagra, while he may have lost interest and simply refuses to do so. These situations can clearly create conflicts, and in these settings, the couple should attempt to address their respective needs openly and candidly; if that fails, they may need to seek professional counseling.

Margery Eagan, a Boston-based journalist who writes a weekly column for the *Boston Herald* newspaper, recently addressed this issue— the impact of Viagra on older couples—this way: "Sex pill is making men happy, but some women are singing the blues." Overall, the column was hilarious: Ms. Eagan referred to "long-suffering Florida wives who now face a grim choice: endure their drug-restored delusional stallion, or risk his sailing into the sunset with a spring-chicken, 45-year-old!" But real-life couples have confirmed for us that it's hardly that way. To the contrary, the couples with whom we have spoken confirmed, in each case, that so far the use of Viagra has enabled them to re-activate their stalled sex lives. Still, Eagan posed a serious long-term question: "Are we really smarter than Mother Nature?" She resorted to Plato's *Republic, Book I*: "Take the poet Sophocles, for example, I was with him once, when someone asked him: 'How do you stand, Sophocles, in respect to the pleasures of sex? Are you still capable of intercourse?' 'Hush sir,' he said. 'It gives me the greatest of joy to have escaped the clutches of that savage and fierce master.'"

Lastly, partners may also occasionally find themselves asking: Is it me—my attractiveness, my sexuality—or is it simply the fact that my partner is "on the pill?" Interestingly enough, for example, many women whose husbands are now in their fifties and sixties are also the first generation of women who were sexually "liberated," themselves, by the introduction of the birth control pill. Then, women suddenly found themselves free to make sexual choices as they never had before—the dark fear of an unwanted pregnancy no longer hung over their heads. A whole new perspective was introduced into many relationships and marriages; with the availability of birth control pills, women could feel free to have sex whenever they chose—and with whomever they chose.

Will Viagra have the same effect in relationships? Now, many men who suffer from E.D. can seek treatment. Still, you should keep in mind that Viagra, plain and simply, does *not* work—i.e., cause an erection— unless some degree of sexual stimulation is present. A partner still has a pivotal role in helping his or her partner achieve an erection. As such, Viagra should simply be viewed as a medication that helps facilitate an erection, so attractiveness and sexuality of the partner remain a key component, even when using Viagra.

WHY SO MUCH HOOPLA WITH VIAGRA?

As a communications professional who has worked in the health care arena for twenty-five years, I've witnessed a lot of "breakthrough" and/or hot medical news stories, of one kind or another. Who can forget the fanfare and excitement, for example, when Prozac® was approved by the FDA for treatment of garden-variety depression, or the fear and upset all of us felt when the first news reports of a lethal, heretofore unknown virus—HIV—trickled in during the early 1980s? Or the interest and hope we felt when Redux®, a new treatment for obesity, entered the market? Still, the media attention that both Redux and Prozac received, in my opinion, pales in comparison to the media frenzy swirling around Viagra. I asked my two male co-authors what they thought about this; I was curious to see if their views were the same as mine. Suffice it to say, their respective responses boiled down to this: Viagra's about men and sex, and *any* talk about sex will pretty much get a man's attention.

Dr. Kloner then sent me an article from the *Los Angeles Times*, "Viagra Users Not Looking Before Leaping," by Martin Miller. In this piece, Miller raised the question of whether the fear of side effects due to Viagra might slow down men from seeking it, but he concluded that the answer is a resounding no! Although the American Academy of Ophthalmology issued a brief statement in mid-May regarding potential eye problems due to the use of Viagra, the side effect of changes in vision, such as seeing a bluish tinge for several hours after taking the drug, did not seem to slow down the number of men seeking prescriptions. Neither have the other minor side effects, including reports of headaches, dizzy spells, and/or indigestion. In fact, one UCLA urologist that Miller wrote to, said "there's been no slowdown in patients wanting prescriptions . . . I've written several hundred prescriptions so far and I haven't heard one complaint."

Miller also chatted with local Los Angeles psychologists, who essentially concluded that sex was so important to men that "there's only one side effect that would scare men off Viagra—death!" One psychologist quoted in the article said this: "Look at how many men play Russian roulette with their lives already for sex . . . There are life-threatening diseases out there, and many don't stop to put on a condom. . . . Anyone who thinks that a few little side effects are going to stop men from seeking pleasure should have their heads examined."

Still, through July 1998, sixty-nine men in the U.S. using Viagra have died, but these deaths have not seemed to slow sales of Viagra. Thus, it looks like Viagra is here to stay—and, with it, a new day dawns on many adult sexual relationships.

—ANN M. HOLMES

How Will Viagra Affect Relationships if It Has a Beneficial Effect in Women?

At this time, Viagra is under clinical investigation in women. Its use may result in increased lubrication and/or better orgasms in women. This is possible because during sexual activity, the clitoris becomes engorged with blood, as does a man's penis. Thus, it is possible that by enhancing clitoral engorgement with Viagra, an orgasm will be achieved or enhanced during sexual activity. To date, the results of ongoing trials are not yet known.

If Viagra is effective in women, then again, it may help to improve a couple's relationship and enhance their mutual pleasure. More will be known about Viagra and women after the clinical studies are completed.

Viagra in Gay Men

Viagra is effective in many men with E.D.—gay, bisexual, or hetero-sexual—and therefore its appropriate use may improve their relation-ships as well. There are early reports that it is being used in gay men with success.

Again, a word of caution here for gay men who use amyl nitrite or amyl nitrate (so-called "poppers") to enhance sexual experience. These agents are organic nitrates, and as we made clear in Chapter 7, Viagra is 100 percent contraindicated in anyone taking organic nitrates. A severe drop in blood pressure, loss of consciousness, heart attack, or even death can occur when Viagra is taken with any nitrate formulation. Simply stated, organic nitrates and Viagra *do not* mix.

Viagra and Behavior: Are There Other Effects?

Finally, one might ask: could Viagra induce a man to commit rape? We feel strongly that anyone who uses a medication is still 100 percent re-sponsible for his own behavior.

To be sure, we think Viagra is here to stay, and even newer, more effective oral medications are likely in the offing. As such, couples need to be aware that these new medications can change the way we think about our sexual health and wellness.

9

What Next On the Horizon for Viagra?

Simply stated, virtually any time a new, promising drug is introduced, hope springs eternal. Remember Redux, for example? No sooner was the drug on the market for the management of clinical obesity (*i.e.*, defined as at least 25 percent above desired body weight) than hundreds of thousands of patients obtained prescriptions, many of them simply to lose ten pounds or so. However, less than eighteen months after FDA approval, the FDA directed the manufacturer to withdraw the drug from the market because studies showed that the drug could damage heart valves. Then, an avalanche of lawsuits followed; today, some estimates put the drug manufacturer's liabilities upwards of $4.5 billion! As you can imagine, Redux gave new meaning to the phrase, a "crash and burn" pharmaceutical product. On the other hand, another drug that was introduced several years ago—Prozac—also took physicians and patients alike by storm when it entered the market, but Prozac has fared quite well, and for more than eight years. Many of the patients who were given Prozac as soon as it became available quickly reported relief from depression. Shortly thereafter, the makers of Prozac, the Indianapolis-based giant Eli Lilly & Co., began to carry out additional clinical studies to see if Prozac might be effective in other mental disorders, in addition to depression. Sure enough, the results of trials showed that Prozac could also provide relief for obsessive-compulsive disorder, panic attacks, and other maladies. To date, it's fair to say that there's been very little disappointment with Prozac and its sister drugs, Zoloft and Paxil.

Still, what these examples illustrate is that drug development is a *very* high-risk business. It takes years of research, followed by years of studies to determine whether a drug will be both safe and effective enough in treating a particular disorder or disease to receive approval from the FDA. Within the first four months on the market, there is already some controversy regarding the use of Viagra. Among about 2.5 million men on the drug, there were sixty-nine deaths. However, twelve were associated with nitrate use and the other cases were likely associated with heart disease. Again, we suggest that patients with heart disease discuss both sexual activity and the use of Viagra with their physicians. Sexual activity alone is associated with a small but finite risk of having a cardiac event.

Viagra in Women

Now, on to use of Viagra in women. Clearly, the Viagra studies have shown how effective and useful it is in a wide range of men, aged nineteen to eighty-seven years, some of whom had diabetes, others who had hypertension, still others had a history of prostrate surgery or spinal cord injury. So far, men who are prescribed Viagra continue to report that they find it safe, effective, and useful in renewing their intimate relationships. So, where will Viagra go from here? One logical next step to pursue in the scientific and medical investigation of Viagra, of course, is to explore whether it will have any beneficial effects in women.

Will Viagra work for women? Before we can answer this question, we need to ask: "What *is* sexual dysfunction in women?" Unfortunately, there are fewer studies in the literature on female sexual dysfunction than male dysfunction. In addition, male sexual dysfunction, especially E.D., is reasonably easy to assess. But what constitutes female sexual dysfunction? Dr. Irwin Goldstein, professor of urology at Boston University School of Medicine, includes the following items as suggestive of female sexual dysfunction, as described in a recent *New York Times* story by Gina Kolata in April 1998:

- discomfort during sexual intercourse
- vaginal dryness
- prolonged time for sexual arousal to occur
- decreased ability to attain orgasm
- diminished clitoral sensation

In another *New York Times* article, Kolata reported that in one survey of 300 adult women, Goldstein found that, overall, 58 percent of the women were affected by female sexual dysfunction, according to the criteria listed here. Sexual dysfunction was most common among older women and in those with vascular disease (just as in the finding in men). Of course, as women age and pass through menopause, they are more prone to vascular and heart disease, and the vasculature of the female sexual organs is not spared by aging and atherosclerotic changes. As such, a decrease in delivery of blood to the sexual organs can occur and contribute to female sexual dysfunction.

Loss of desire for sexual activity is another factor that may play an important role, especially as women age. However, physical factors such as decrease in vaginal lubrication and decrease in arousal may also contribute to loss of desire.

In order to test the efficacy of a drug developed to improve sexual function in women, an appropriate questionnaire needs to be developed. Because the female sexual response differs in many ways from the male's response, the questionnaire is likely to look quite different from the one used for men—the IIEF questionnaire or scale, described in Chapter 5. Questionnaires for female sexual dysfunction are currently being developed by Pfizer Inc, the manufacturer of Viagra, in anticipation of further research into female sexual dysfunction.

Are there other modalities we could use to measure female sexual dysfunction? Again, Gina Kolata reported in April 1998 in the *New York Times* that Dr. Raymond Rosen of the Robert Wood Johnson Medical School in New Jersey tested Vasomax (phentolamine) in six women who had difficulties with sexual arousal. When they watched a pornographic movie after taking the medicine, blood flow to the vagina increased as recorded by a special tampon, capable of measuring blood flow. In association with the measured blood flow, the women reported a feeling of increased vaginal wetness and a "pleasant tingling sensation" of their genitals, a feeling that was not present without the phentolamine.

Other techonology might measure clitoral tumescence, which is the parallel phenomenon of male erection. It is likely that now that such drugs as phentolamine (Vasomax) and sildenafil (Viagra) have been developed, there will be much more research into female sexual dysfunction and treatment. Until very recently, therapies for sexual dysfunction in men and women have been lacking, but especially for women. Hormone

---

CASE #1: HAPPINESS IS . . .

Paula and Mark have been married for twenty-seven years, "virtually all of them good years," Mark says with a chuckle. But shortly after Mark turned sixty, he experienced a decline in his ability to have an erection satisfactory for sexual intercourse. Fortunately, he and his wife Paula were able to talk about the problem openly, but Mark did not want to see a physician. Paula decided to take matters into her own hands; at her annual checkup with her ob-gyn, she told him about Mark's difficulties and asked him for advice. He referred the couple to Dr. Jarow. Mark was reluctant to seek medical help, but Paula persuaded him that it was worth a try. After completing the IIEF questionnaire, Mark and Paula met with Dr. Jarow and talked over their responses. Dr. Jarow conducted a physical exam and ordered basic laboratory tests. Mark had high blood pressure and was treated for it, along with the E.D. On a recent followup visit, Dr. Jarow said, Mark grinned from ear to ear when asked how he and Paula were doing with Viagra. "It's so easy," Mark responds, "I feel like a young man again. We're both so grateful!"

---

replacement therapy is available for women; estrogens reduce problems such as atrophic vaginitis, and there are a whole host of lubricating jellies available, too, for this condition. These treatments, however, do not treat the root of the female sexual dysfunction.

Should medications such as Viagra and Vasomax work? Will improving blood flow to female genitalia improve sexual function and satisfaction? While the exact answers to these questions are still not known, there is reason to be guardedly optimistic. To begin with, both male and female sexual organs share many parallel structures. Hormones expressed during fetal development turn certain embryonic structures into either the male or female equivalent. The most notable example is the female clitoris, which shares certain properties with the penis. Like the penis, it becomes engorged with blood during sexual arousal, and it has a similar distribution of nerves. The female vulva parallels the male scrotum; the testes, in turn, parallel the ovaries. Theoretically, Viagra should increase blood flow to the clitoris during sexual activity because female genitalia also contain PDE_5, the enzyme Viagra inhibits. By increasing blood flow to the clitoris, Viagra may enhance sexual arousal, sensitivity, and improve the ability to have orgasms. If Viagra improves blood flow to the vagina, it theoretically may improve vaginal lubrication.

Pfizer currently is conducting two Phase II studies out of one of their main research facilities in Sandwich to address the issue of whether or not Viagra will improve female sexual function. To date, hundreds of women in several cities throughout Europe are involved in these studies. At present, results from these studies are not expected until the end of 1998 or perhaps early 1999. In addition, there are some independent researchers who are also conducting their own studies.

Lastly, although we know that at the time of this writing there have been sixty-nine reported deaths among about 2.5 million men who used Viagra, we still have *no* idea whether there are the same and/or additional safety issues in women. Theoretically, any woman taking nitrates for heart disease could also have precipitous drops in blood pressure if she also took Viagra. An additional concern is what Viagra might do to human pregnancies. While pregnant animals did not develop problems with Viagra, and there was no teratogenic effects among the births, there is simply no data on the effect of Viagra in pregnant women.

Media reports have also described women who have asked their physicians to write them a prescription for Viagra. In some cases, the physicians are doing so. Such off-labeling prescribing is a medical decision that can be made by an individual physician. For example, many drugs are approved for one or more uses but are still prescribed for additional uses. However, until we have more data on the effect of Viagra in women, including possible risks, widespread prescribing of the drug for women is probably inadvisable.

Couples on Viagra

As we discussed in earlier chapters, many couples have reported that due to the use of Viagra, their sex lives—and their level of shared emotional intimacy—has improved (see Case #1 and Case #2 in this chapter). For those men in whom Viagra is effective, it does seem that the benefits of taking the drug far outweigh the side effects (again, a reminder that taking Viagra with nitrates is contraindicated). But apparently, use of Viagra occasionally results in disrupting a relationship, too. It didn't take long, for example, for lawyers to seize the opportunity to represent one or more women who claim that their mates (in some cases, husbands, and in other cases, live-in mates), left them, apparently due to the effects that Viagra had on their psyche. In one case that we know of, for example, a well-to-do Long Island man left his live-in companion of more than five years. Why? According to the attorney representing her—and he claims to be representing other women sharing a similar plight—her mate had been impotent for several years, but after taking Viagra, he was able to experience successful sexual intercourse. Very soon thereafter, he decided that the grass might be greener elsewhere and he left, apparently in hot pursuit of those greener pastures (it was reported he moved in with another woman). According to the lawyer, he simply left a note in the household for her instructing her to keep the property, the bank account, and the Mercedes—he was off to a new life!

To begin with, it certainly remains to be seen whether that man will enjoy a "new" or better life. Keep in mind, as we've said throughout this book, that E.D. is a medical condition—one that can, and often does—have an adverse effect on one's quality of life. If this man determined that, with his restored erectile function, he now had an increased opportunity to achieve a better quality of life for himself, than that is his decision. Despite what may have occurred in this one reported case, we don't think it is likely that anyone will successfully be able to blame appropriate use of a medication for the collapse of their personal life.

And what about the possibility of women approaching physicians to obtain Viagra for their partners, even though neither they nor their partners have a specific complaint of E.D.? Some women have revealed they hoped their partners would become a "super-stud" by taking Viagra. Again, the concern here is that men with normal erections should not take this medication in order to become a "sexual superman," especially if E.D. is not present. Viagra is only indicated for men with E.D., and it should only be used as indicated.

Coping with Insurance: Who Pays for Viagra?

Managed-care organizations, insurance companies, and patient advocates alike are still very busy tackling this question. In general, managed-care organizations want to satisfy their patient-consumer demands, but they also don't want to lose money in the process. For example, according to one recent account in the *San Francisco Chronicle*, it was estimated that a very large managed-care organization such as Kaiser Permaneate of Northern California could spend as much as fifty million dollars a year dispensing Viagra at $7 per pill to patients who needed it. As of June

CASE #2: MAKING A COMEBACK WITH VIAGRA!

Jack C. worked hard his whole life; by the time he was forty-two years old, he was well on his way to a very successful career. He enjoyed his children and had a stable marriage, too. "Everything was fine," he remarked, "until I reached my fiftieth birthday." As Jack tells it, from that time on, things just "began to unravel." What happened? For starters, Jack developed prostate cancer; he had surgery, was relieved to be rid of the cancer, and then found himself stuck with another disorder: E.D. Slowly, he and his wife drifted apart; Jack simply felt at a loss and did not know what to do. During this time, he met another woman, and he decided to see a urologist to see what could be done about his E.D. Dr. Jarow evaluated him and treated him with a vacuum pump, since little else was available at that time. A year or two later, Jack developed Peyronie's disease, and Dr. Jarow performed surgery to correct the problem. Dr. Jarow didn't see Jack again until very recently, when he came in for an appointment, this time looking for Viagra. "It's incredible," he said. "We both feel great knowing I have this medication to use." His long-term affair continues; he has not had a sexual relationship with his wife, he has told us, since the prostate surgery more than a decade ago.

Interestingly enough, we include this case to show you some of the issues physicians face when prescribing medication. In this instance, Dr. Jarow felt it was his responsibility to provide appropriate medical treatment for a patient seeking it; he did not attempt marital counseling.

1998, Kaiser announced that they will not cover the cost of Viagra. At present, there isn't any consensus among managed-care organizations on reimbursement for Viagra, although there is no question that patients are demanding it.

The real issue for these organizations, then, is whether they should pay for so-called "lifestyle" medicines. These medicines may improve overall health, well-being, and quality of life but are not necessarily a "medical necessity." In other words, if your HMO won't give you a "quality-of-life medicine," you aren't likely to drop dead because of it. Examples of "lifestyle medicines" include drugs such as topical minoxidil for baldness, the oral pill Propecia for baldness, Retin-A for diminishing wrinkles, plastic surgery for reducing wrinkles, and even diet pills. We are not aware of anyone who has become gravely ill due to baldness or wrinkled skin. Of course, if someone is morbidly obese, an insurance company might cover diet pills, but modestly obese individuals generally are not likely to be covered.

Some managed-care organizations are considering adding a type of "lifestyle" benefit package that would include some of the medicines mentioned here, as well as items such as cosmetic surgery and even alternative medicine. This type of package, however, will add costs for the consumer.

So, where are the HMOs to date on Viagra? In California, some managed-care organizations will pay for Viagra (limiting prescriptions to six pills per month) when E.D. is diagnosed and clearly is due to an underlying medical problem, such as diabetes, prostrate surgery, or a neurologic condition. Pacificare, another HMO in California, does not currently cover Viagra but does cover penile injection therapy, whereas HealthNet is still studying the issue of reimbursement for Viagra. (HealthNet does cover injections and alprostadil suppositories.) Blue Shield's AccessPlus HMO will likely cover Viagra when it is due to specific medical problems. CIGNA Healthcare also requires documented organic E.D. due to a treated medical condition in order to cover Viagra. It also has a six-tablet-per-month limit. Lastly, in New York City, a $10 million lawsuit was filed against the Oxford Healthcare Plan by a diabetic man who wants coverage for his Viagra. At the time of this writing, decisions by many of these companies are pending or may change.

How does Viagra stack up vis-a-vis birth control pills? If an HMO decides to cover Viagra, but does not cover birth control pills, does this mean that the HMO is running the risk of a discrimination lawsuit? For the HMOs previously mentioned that cover oral contraceptives, ultimately, Viagra may get covered, too.

Finally, it does appear that even if HMOs and insurance companies continue to tighten their coverage policies of Viagra, many men, in fact, might be willing to pay "out-of-pocket" for Viagra. We recently saw estimates that put the percentage of men who are paying for Viagra by themselves—without reimbursement from insurers—at about 50 percent. As insurers tighten restrictions, this percentage may increase. However, it is unlikely that sales of Viagra will drop because of rules from HMOs and insurance companies.

Let's face it: sex sells!

And Medicaid?

Will government programs such as Medicaid pay for Viagra? In May 1998, the White House instructed state officials to require their respective Medicaid programs to cover the costs of Viagra. Like the HMOs and other insurers, it is likely that the states will limit the number of pills per month that they cover. Up until now some states did cover costs of Viagra, others did not, and still others were studying the issue. When state Medicaid programs cover prescription drugs, they are required to follow federal regulations and cannot arbitrarily omit certain drugs. Drugs such as birth control pills, which fall under the category of "family-planning services and supplies" currently are covered under federal Medicaid laws.

A spokesman for Pfizer Inc stated that Medicaid coverage for Viagra was justifiable, given the fact that many states already pay for other types of E.D. therapies, such as MUSE and injections, which are much more expensive. Finally, the federal government's Medicare program covers only in-patient prescription drugs; the question of whether to cover Viagra has not been an issue.

Global Lust for Viagra: News from Around the World

Despite the reports of more than sixty deaths, sales of Viagra have not slowed in the U.S., nor has interest in the product declined globally—to the contrary, in fact, although as of this writing the drug has only been approved for use in the U.S., and a few Latin American countries; approval is expected in at least another thirty countries by the end of 1999. In fact, the European Union (fifteen member countries) gave its blessing to Viagra in mid-September 1998; member countries should have the drug available for patients by October or November 1998. In addition, the black market already is in full-swing; specifically, one report we know of suggests that you can obtain Viagra in Italy—although it's not approved there yet—for $50 per pill! Other reports say men are flying from country to country to obtain Viagra, either legitimately—*i.e.*, in a country where Viagra is approved for use—or illegitimately, in a country where the black market for the drug is flourishing. Much smaller states, for example, such as San Marino and Andorra, have been over-run by men visiting simply to obtain Viagra! From Taiwan to Turkey, men seem willing to pay anywhere from

$60 to $800 per bottle, black market prices! Unfortunately, it does seem that some of these men mistakenly believe that Viagra will enhance their sexual prowess; again, that is simply not so. Viagra is a medical treatment, developed to help men with E.D. achieve erections satisfactory for sexual intercourse. Adequate sexual stimulation also must occur. To think that, even for a moment, Viagra will turn a man into a "sexual superman" is ridiculous! Nevertheless, we have heard reports that some men abroad believe this is true, a tale that is no doubt fueled by the black marketeers.

We believe that much of this activity will come to a halt because the European Agency for the Evaluation of Medicinal Products has adopted a "positive opinion" on Viagra. Thus, Viagra is likely to be available quite soon in the fifteen-country region.

Finally, when sixteen deaths were reported in the U.S. in men who were taking Viagra, Vietnam decided to ban sales of the drug—at least for the time being. Officials say they need more information before they change course on the drug. Israel has recently lifted a ban it had imposed on Viagra.

Cultural Considerations

Will Viagra necessarily fare better in other Western countries, where men and women tend to be more open about discussing sex? At this early stage, it's really anyone's best guess, but so far, Viagra is only available in a few Latin American countries, countries in which "male macho" reigns supreme. We anticipate that the drug will sell well in all of these countries. Also, it's possible that since sex is one of the very few free *and* pleasurable events left in life, the drug may enjoy an unusually high rate of early acceptance worldwide, regardless of religion, culture, or socioeconomic status. Clearly, more will be known about global acceptance and use as Viagra is approved and used in more and more countries around the world.

What else can we say about Viagra? Now, only time will tell; the Viagra story continues to unfold before us. But we believe one thing is clear: Viagra represents an end, as well as a beginning. For many men, Viagra holds the promise of ending their experiences with E.D., and allowing them the opportunity to begin to recapture their sexual health and wellness. In the final analysis, restoring health and wellness is always what good medicine is all about.

Bibliography

American Heart Association, 1998 Heart and Strokes Statistical Update. Dallas, Texas. American Heart Association Monograph, 1997.

Althof, S.E. and Seftel, A.D.. "The evaluation and management of erectile dysfunction." Clinical Sexuality. *Psychiat Clin North Amer.* 18 (1995) 171–192.

Azadzoi, K.M., Siroky, M.G., Goldstein, I. "Study of etiologic relationship of arterial atherosclerosis to corporal veno-occlusive dysfunction in the rabbit." *J Urol.* 155 (1996) 1745–1800.

Ballard, S.A., Gingell, C.J.C., Price, M.E. et al. "Sildenafil, an inhibitor of phophodiesderase type 5, enhances nitric oxide mediated relaxation of human corpus cavernosum." *Int J Impot Res.* 8 (1996) 103.

Baum, N., Rhodes, D. "A practical approach to the evaluation and treatment of erectile dysfunction. A private practitioner's viewpoint." *Urol Clin North Amer.* 22 (1995) 865–877.

Becker, A.J., Stief, C.G., Schultheiss, D. et al. "Double blind study on oral phentolamine as treatment for ED. " Abstract. *J Urol.* 159 (1997) 202.

Benson, G.S., Boileau, M.A. "The penis: sexual function and dysfunction." In: Gillenwater, J.Y., Grayhack, J.T., Howards, S.S., Duckett, J.W., eds. *Adult and Pediatric Urology.* 3rd ed. Mosby: St. Louis, Mo. 1996:1951–1993.

Boolell, M., Allen, M.J., Ballard, S.A. et al. "Sildenafil: an orally active type 5 cyclic GMP-specific phosphodiesterase inhibitor for the treatment of penile E.D." *Int J Impot Res.* 8 (1996) 47–52.

Boolell, M., Gepi-Attee, S., Gingell, J.C., Allen, M.J. "Sildenafil, a novel effective oral therapy for male E.D." *Br J Urol.* 78 (1996) 257–261.

Boolell, M., Gepi-Attee, S., Gingell, C. "UK-92, 480: a new oral treatment for E.D. A double-blind, placebo controlled crossover study demonstrating dose response with Rigiscan and efficacy with outpatient diary." Abstract. *Urology.* 155 (supplement) (1996) 495A.

Boolell, M., Pearsen, J., Gingell, J.C. et al. "Sildenafil (VIAGRA™) is an efficacious oral therapy in diabetic patients with E.D. (ED). *Int J Impot Res.* 8 (1996) 186.

Boolell, M., Yates, P.K., Wulff, M.B. et al. "Sildenafil (VIAGRA™) A new oral treatment with rapid onset of action for penile E.D. (ED)." *Int J Impot Res.* 8 (1996) 47–52

Bronowski, J. *Science and Human Values.* Harper & Row: New York, NY (1956).

Burnett, A.L. "Role of nitric oxide in the physiology of erection." *Biol Reprod.* 52 (1995) 485–489.

Burnett, A.L. "Nitric oxide in the penis: physiology and pathology." *J Urol.* 157 (1997) 320–324.

Buvat, J., Gingell, C.J., Jardin, A. et al. "Sildenafil (VIAGRA™) an oral treatment for E.D: a 1 year, open-label, extension study." *Urology.* Abstract. (1997)

Christ, G.J. "The penis as a vascular organ. The importance of corporal smooth muscle tone in the control of erection." *Urol Clin North Amer.* 22 (1995) 727–745.

Christiansen, E. and the Multicentre Study Group. "Sildenafil (VIAGRA™) A new oral treatment for E.D. (ED): Results of a 16 week open dose escalation study." *Int J Impot Res.* 8 (1996) 147.

Comroe, Julius H. Jr., *Retrospectroscope: Insights into Medical Discovery.* Van Gehr Press: Menlo Park, Cal (1977).

Cuzin, B., Emrich, H.M., Meuleman, E.J.H. et al. "Sildenafil (VIAGRA™): a 6-month, double-blind, placebo-controlled, flexible dose escalation study in patients with E.D." Abstract; in press. *Int J Impot Res.* (1998).

Daily News Staff and Wire. "Deaths reported by Pfizer. Six Viagra patients die; shares stumble." *Los Angeles Daily News.* May 23, 1998.

Data on file, Pfizer Inc, New York, NY.

Dear, R. "White House plans medicaid coverage of Viagra by states." *New York Times.* May 27, 1998.

Dinsmore, W.W., Gingell, C.J., Jardin, A. et al. "Sildenafil (VIAGRA™). A new oral treatment for E.D. (ED). A double-blind, placebo-controlled, parallel group, once daily dose response study." *Int J Impot Res.* 8 (1996) 147.

Eardley, I., Morgan, R.S., Dinsmore, W.W. "UK-92, 480: a new oral therapy for E.D., a double-blind, placebo controlled trial with treatment taken as required." Abstract. *Urology.* (1996).

El-Sukka, A.I., Lue, T.F. "Does a heart attack mean the end of sexual life? American College of Cardiology Educational Highlights/Winter" (1996) 6–9.

FDA website, August 24, 1998.

Feldman, H.A., Goldstein, I., Hatzichristou, D.G., Krane, R.J., McKinlay, J.B., "Impotence and its medical and psychological correlates: results of the Massachusetts Male Aging Study." *J Urol.* 151 (1994) 54–61.

Gardner, B.P., Glass, C., Fraser, M. et al. "Sildenafil (VIAGRA™). A double-blind, placebo-controlled, single dose, two-way crossover study in men with E.D. caused by traumatic spinal cord injury." Abstract. *Urology*. (1996).

GCP, Good Clinical Practices. Barton Polansky Association, Inc. October 1995.

Gingell, C.J.C., Jordan, A., Olsson, A.M. et al. "UK-92, 480. A new oral treatment for E.D.: A double-blind, placebo-controlled, once daily dose response study." Abstract. *Urology*. 155 (supplement): 495A. (1996).

Goldstein, I., Lue, T.F., Padma-Nathan, H. et al., for the Sildenafil Study Group. "Oral sildenafil in the treatment of Erectile dysfunction." *N Engl J Med*. 338 (1998) 1397–1404.

Greenstein, A., Chen, J., Miller, H., et al. "Does severity of ischemic coronary disease correlate with erectile function?" *Int J Impot Re*. 9 (1997) 123–126.

Handy, B. "The Viagracraze." *Time* (May 4, 1998) 50–57.

Hedley, W.S. "Roentgen rays. A survey, present and retrospective." *Arch Roentgen Ray*. 2 (1897) 6–12.

"HMO's fear cost of new drugs, Viagra, others may put plans in financial bind." *San Francisco Chronicle*. May 25, 1998.

Hutter, A.M., Cheitlin, M.D. et al. ACC/AHA Summary Statement on the Use of Sildenafil (Viagra™) in patients at Clinical Risk from Cardiovascular Effects, August 10, 1998.

Ignarro, L.J., Lippton, H., Edwards, J.C., et al. "Mechanism of vascular smooth muscle relaxation by organic nitrates, nitrites, nitroprusside and nitric oxide: evidence for the involvement of S-nitrosothiols as active intermediates." *J Pharmacol Exp Ther*. 218 (1981) 739–749.

Jaffe, A., Chen, Y., Kisch, E.S., et al. "Erectile dysfunction in hypertensive subjects. Assessment of potential determinants." *Hypertension*. 28 (1996) 859–862.

Kaiser, F.E. "Sexuality in the elderly." *Urol Clin North Amer*. 23 (1996) 99–109.

Klein, R., Klein, B.E.K., Lee, K.E., et al. "Prevalence of self-reported erectile dysfunction in people with long-term IDDM. *Diabetes Care*." 19 (1996) 135–141.

Kolata, G. "New drug for impotence raises hope for its use by women, too." *New York Times*. April 4, 1998.

Kolata, G. "Doctors debate use of drug to help women's sex lives." *New York Times*. April 25, 1998.

Linet, O.I., Ogrina FG. Efficacy and safety of intracavernosal alprostadil in men with E.D." *N Engl J Med*. 334 (1996) 873–877.

Lue, T.F., and the Sildenafil Study Group. "A study of sildenafil (VIAGRA™) a new oral agent for the treatment of male E.D." *Abstract. Urology*. 1997.

Lue, T.F., Broderick, G. "Evaluation and nonsurgical management of erectile dysfunction and priapism." In: Walsh, P.C., ed. *Campbell's Urology.* Volume 2, 7th ed. Saunders, Philadelphia, PA. (1998) 1181–1207.

Lugnier, C., Komas, N. "Modulation of vascular cyclic nucleotide phosphodiesterases by cyclic GMP: role in vasodilatation. *Eur Heart J.* 14 (supplement 1) (1993) 141–148.

McConnell, J.D., Wilson, J.D. Impotence. In: Fauci, A.S. et. al, eds. *Harrison's Principles of Internal Medicine.* 14th ed. New York, NY McGraw-Hill Book Company (1998) 286–289.

Montorsi, F., Morgan, R.J., Olsoson, A.M. et al. "Sildenafil (VIAGRA™): a 3-month, double-blind, placebo-controlled, fixed dose study in patients with E.D." (supplement) In press. *Eur Urol.* (1998)

Morley, J.E. "Impotence." *Am J Med.* 80 (1986) 897–905.

Morley, J.E., Kaiser, F.E. "Sexual function with advancing age. Geriatric medicine in Medical Clinics of North America." 73 (1989)1483–1495.

Moss, H.B., Procci, W.R. "Sexual dysfunction associated with oral antihypertensive medication: A critical survey of the literature." *Gen Hosp Psychiat.* 4 (1982) 121–129.

Muirhead, G.J., Allen, M.J., James, G.C. et al. "Pharmacokinetics of sildenafil (VIAGRA™), a selective cGMP PDE$_5$ inhibitor, after single oral dose in fasted and healthy volunteers." Proceedings of the British Pharmacological Society University of Leicester UK. 2 (August 1996) 268.

Muller, J.E., Mittleman, M.A., Maclure, M. et al. "Triggering Myocardial Infarction by Sexual Activity." *JAMA* 275 (1996) 1405–1409.

Muller, S.C., El-Damanhoury, E.L., Ruth, J., et al. "Hypertension and impotence." *Eur Urol.* 19 (1991) 29–34.

Mulligan, T., Katz, P.G. "Why aged men become impotent." *Arch Intern Med.* 149 (1989) 1365–1366.

NIH Consensus Conference Development Panel on Impotence. "Impotence." *JAMA.* 270 (1993) 83–90.

Padma-Nathan, H., Hellstrom, W.J.G., Kaiser, F.E. et al. "Treatment of men with E.D. with transurethral alprostadil." *N Engl J Med.* 336 (1997) 1–7.

Pierson, Ransdell. "Viagra sales seen zooming despite insurer curbs." *Reuters News Service.* April 29, 1998.

Rosen, R.C., Riley, A., Wagner, G., Osterloh, I.H., Kirkpatrick, J., Mishna, A. "The International Index of Erectile Function (IIEF): a multidimensional scale for assessment of E.D." *Urology* 49 (1997) 822–830.

Rowland, H.A., Thomson, B., Pupin, M.I., Kennelly, A.B. "The Röntgen ray and its relation to physics: a topical discussion." *Trans Amer Inst Elect Engin.* 13 (1896) 403–432.

Sheridan, M.B. "Men around the globe lust after Viagra." *Los Angeles Times.* May 26, 1998.

Sherman, W. "Now woman catch love-drug bug." *New York Post.* (month day),1998.

Spear, F.G. "Early days of experimental radiology." *Br J Radiol.* 46 (1973) 762–765.

Terrett, N.R., Bell, A.S., Brown, D., Ellis, P. "Sildenafil (VIAGRA™), a potent and selective inhibitor of type 5 cGMP phophodiesterase with utility for the treatment of male E.D." *Bioorg Medicin Chem Let.* 6 (1996) 1819–1824.

Thompson, S. "First presidential address to the Roentgen Society." *Arch Roentgen Ray.* 2 (1897) 23–30.

Utiger, R.D. "A pill for impotence." Editorial. *N Engl J Med.* 338 (1998) 1458–1459.

Viagra™ (sildenafil citrate). Prescribing information. Pfizer Inc: New York, NY. (1998).

Virag, R., Bouilly, P., Frydman, D. "Is impotence an arterial disorder? A study of arterial risk factors in 440 impotent men." *Lancet.* 8422 (1985) 181–184.

Wassertheill-Smaller, S., Blaufox, M.D., Oberman, A., et al. "Effect of antihypertensives on sexual function and quality of life: The TAIM Study." *Ann Intern Med.* 114 (1991) 613–620.

Wei, M., Macera, C.A., Davis, D.R., et al. "Total cholesterol and high density lipoprotein cholesterol as important predicators of erectile dysfunction." *Am J Epidemiol.* 140 (1994) 930–937.

Zorgniotti, A.W. "Experience with buccal phentolamine mesylate for impotence." *Int J Impot Res.* 6 (1994) 37–41.

Index

P

Penile implants, 116–117
Performance anxiety, 123
Peyronie's disease, 53
Pfizer, Inc., 71, 75, 79, 126, 133, 134
Physicians
  to consult about E.D. (erectile dysfunction), 44–45
  and describing your E.D. (erectile dysfunction), 54
  evaluation of patient, 49–50
  and lab studies, 61
  and nocturnal erections assessment, 62–63
  and patient consultation, 45–48
  and patient history, 52–53
  and physical exam, 59–60
  and vascular evaluation, 61–62
Premature ejaculation, 53
Prolactin, 35
Prostheses, 117
Provim, 112–113
Psychological
  effects of Viagra, 123–125
  origins of E.D. (erectile dysfunction), 21

R

Retarded ejaculation, 53
Rosen, Raymond, 133

S

Scientific discovery, in general, 71–75
Sexual Health Inventory for Men (IIEF-5), 69–70
Sexually transmitted diseases, 108
Smoking, 20–21

Spinal cord injuries, 17, 109
Structural abnormalities, 18
Suppositories, 115–116
Surgeries and E.D. (erectile dysfunction), 18, 109–110

T

Testosterone, 34–35
Trazodone (Desyrel), 111
Treatments for E.D. (erectile dysfunction), 51–52, 85, 111–117

V

Vacuum erection device, 114–115
Vascular evaluation, 61–62
Vascular risk factors, 58
Vascular surgery, 116
Vasodilan, 111
Vasomax, 112
Viagra
  and aging, 110
  appropriate use of, 100
  and behavior, 128
  benefits of, 125
  clinical studies of, 90–98, 116
  contraindications to, 103–107
  and coronary heart disease, 107
  and couples, 125–128, 135–136
  and cultural considerations, 140
  and deaths, 114
  and depression, 108, 123–124
  and diabetes, 108
  discovery of, 75–80
  dosage of, 98–100
  and drug interactions, 90, 101–102
  and drug profiles, 87–90
  effectiveness of, 77, 90–98, 98, 110–111